5th Edition

Social Work and Mental Health

Malcolm Golightley

 |

Los Angeles | London | New Delhi
Singapore | Washington DC

Learning Matters
An imprint of SAGE Publications Ltd
1 Oliver's Yard
55 City Road
London EC1Y 1SP

SAGE Publications Inc.
2455 Teller Road
Thousand Oaks, California 91320

SAGE Publications India Pvt Ltd
B 1/I 1 Mohan Cooperative Industrial Area
Mathura Road
New Delhi 110 044

SAGE Publications Asia-Pacific Pte Ltd
3 Church Street
#10–04 Samsung Hub
Singapore 049483

First published in 2004 by Learning Matters Ltd. Reprinted twice in 2005. Second edition published in 2006. Third edition published in 2008. Reprinted in 2009. Fourth edition published in 2011. Fifth edition published in 2014 by SAGE/Learning Matters.

Editor: Luke Block
Production controller: Chris Marke
Project management: Deer Park Productions, Tavistock, Devon
Marketing manager: Tamara Navaratnam
Cover design: Wendy Scott
Typeset by: C&M Digitals (P) Ltd, Chennai, India
Printed by CPI Group (UK) Ltd, Croydon, CR0 4YY

Library of Congress Control Number: 2014930436

British Library Cataloguing in Publication Data

A catalogue record for this book is available from the British Library

MIX
Paper from responsible sources
FSC
www.fsc.org   FSC® C013604

ISBN 978-1-4462-8230-4 (pbk)
ISBN 978-1-4462-8229-8

Contents

List of abbreviations

AC	approved clinician
AMHP	approved mental health professional
ASW	approved social worker; replaced by the AMHP
BASW	British Association of Social Workers
BMA	British Medical Association
BNF	British National Formulary
CAMHS	child and adolescent mental health services
CBT	cognitive behavioural therapy
CMHT	community mental health team
CPA	care programme approach
CPN	community psychiatric nurse
CTO	community treatment order
DoH	Department of Health
DoLS	deprivation of liberty safeguards
EC	European Commission
ECT	electroconvulsive therapy
EE	expressed emotion
GP	general practitioner
HCPC	Health Care Professions Council
MDO	mentally disordered offender
MHT	Mental Health Tribunal
NHS	National Health Service
NMC	Nursing and Midwifery Council
NR	nearest relative (legal term)

OT	occupational therapist
PHCT	primary health care team
RA	Responsible Authority
RMO	responsible medical officer (1983 MHA); now replaced by the RC
RC	responsible clinician
SCIE	Social Care Institute for Excellence
SCT	supervised community treatment
SOAD	second opinion appointed doctor
SSRI	selective serotonin reuptake inhibitor
WHO	World Health Organisation

Acknowledgements

Thanks are due to the countless people who over the years have maintained my interest in mental health. These have been professionals, volunteers, carers and service users. More specifically thanks are due to Professor Bob Peckitt, consultant psychiatrist for advice and guidance for Chapter 2; Christopher Curran, a Fellow of the University of Lincoln, and David Hewitt, a solicitor and Fellow of the University for their considerable expertise and support to help me to unravel the new legislation and Jim Rogers for his help with mental capacity. Thanks must also go to my daughter Sarah who has entered the world of professional social work after a very interesting journey and provides equal measures of advice and love. The popularity of the previous four editions has been as encouraging as it has been a surprise and special thanks need to go to all those students whose praise for the book has been heartwarming and humbling.

This book has been a long time in the making but has allowed me to indulge myself in an area which I am passionate about and have been involved in for over 30 years as a practitioner, academic, researcher, professor and user and carer. I hope the contents do justice to the richness of the experience and to all the things that I have learned from service users and other influential people.

As the number of editions has grown so has my extended family, almost in parallel. While I am not sure what this means it would be very remiss of me not to thank and dedicate this edition to Pam, our family, Sharada and Steve, Rosie and Mathew, Sarah, Liam and my grandchildren Kezie, Harrison, Maddison Rose, Holly May, Wilhem and Bailey.

Introduction

This fifth edition is written with student social workers in mind who are studying for their professional qualifications. While the book is part of a series aimed at an undergraduate level there is no reason that this should not be of interest to postgraduates and students and practitioners of other disciplines.

There are a number of themes that occur throughout the text that form a thread throughout this book but also provide a frame of reference for practice. These are covered briefly now with some signposting for later reading.

First of course is the reality that mental health is everyone's business, so it's no surprise that the most recent policy introduced in July 2012 is called **No Health Without Mental Health** (DoH, 2012). This really does make my first point and that is that mental health is crucial to our wellbeing. The prevalence of mental ill health is such that just about one person in four will at some time in their lives seek help for mental health issues. Sometimes this will be secretive and containable and at other times obvious and indeed in the case of manic-depression (or more accurately bi-polar disorder) the mania phase can give rise to considerable energies and some eminent politicians are thought to have experienced this form of disorder. On other occasions the 'episode' of mental disorder may be so severe that the intervention of professionals is necessary to help the wellbeing of that person or for the protection of others.

A moment's thought about this situation will introduce another of my themes and that is the futility but enduring use of what I term 'binary opposites'. This is the tendency of us all to see people as mad or sane, heterosexual or homosexual polar opposites that deny the reality of everyday life. How many of us can identify people who are 100% sane or 100% mad? It just doesn't work like that! Similarly we search for explanations of mental disorder by looking to medical or social models but these are only compartmentalised for conceptual terms and in no way reflect the reality in which we work and one that has these models with permeable and flexible boundaries. Even the most ardent of biomedical practitioners understands the importance of looking at the whole person. So when we think about these big concepts we might do best by seeing explanations as along a continuum and one that is influenced by time, country and conceptual development.

The third thread goes to the heart of social work as a profession and what I think is the way for the profession to develop over the next decade. Seldom has social work been under so much scrutiny as at present and seldom have the challenges been more profound and so subject to the media spotlight. All of this is also taking place in an era of extreme austerity, evidenced by contracting funding, high workloads and increasing bureaucracy. Government attempts to influence the social work curriculum seem to ignore anything that isn't child protection, until the next mental health crisis. So what is a social worker to do?

One of the most effective ways of working is known as 'psychosocial work' (Coulshed, 1991; Howe, 1998; John and Trevithick, 2012), which enables social workers to bring together a way of working that focuses upon the interplay between the individual's inner world (*psycho*), the very essence of 'metal illness' and the social environment (*socio*). Of course there are other ways of looking at the same situation and taking psychosocial as an approach should not be at the expense of those who see their approach as family therapy, psychoanalytic or indeed radical social work. This in my view and others (Nathan and Webber, 2010,) is at the heart of what we do as social workers. It builds upon a firm tradition of social casework espoused by social work giants such as Hollis, but in recent years the preoccupation has been on what has been called in mental health the 'bureau-medicalisation' of social work practice (Nathan and Webber, 2010). But social work needs, and the grass roots are already showing through, a reaction to this deskilling with a move towards a more therapeutic approach.

At the heart of this approach is what we might all take for granted but which is called relationship working. When we think about 'relational' in respect of social work this is taken to mean a wide range of approaches that start from the very basic of relationships to a therapeutic relationship. This covers the individual's interface with society and others as well as what is happening for the person themselves. The social worker is often faced with challenging situations and, make no mistake, working with people who are very troubled is difficult. The idea of emotional labour helps to explain how the social worker may act as a 'container' in which the strong emotions of the service user are absorbed by the worker.

The importance of relationships as a central tenet of social work practice has long been recognised by leading academics (John and Trevithick, 2003; Howe, 1998; Parton 2008) with Coulshed's seminal work:

> *While it is true that people do not come to social work looking for a relationship, and while it is no substitute for practical support, nevertheless social workers are one of the few groups who recognize the value of relating to others in a way which recognizes their experience as fundamental to understanding and action.*
>
> (Coulshed, 1991, p.2)

These themes will all be built on in the following chapters and I hope that you will see that mental health social work is a very rewarding area to study and to practise.

Requirements for social work education and training

This book has been carefully mapped to the new Professional Capabilities Framework for Social Workers in England and will help you to develop the appropriate standards at the right level. These standards are:

- **Professionalism**

  Identify and behave as a professional social worker committed to professional development.

- **Values and ethics**

  Apply social work ethical principles and values to guide professional practice.

- **Diversity**

  Recognise diversity and apply anti-discriminatory and anti-oppressive principles in practice.

- **Rights, justice and economic wellbeing**

  Advance human rights and promote social justice and economic wellbeing.

- **Knowledge**

  Apply knowledge of social sciences, law and social work practice theory.

- **Critical reflection and analysis**

  Apply critical reflection and analysis to inform and provide a rationale for professional decision-making.

- **Intervention and skills**

  Use judgement and authority to intervene with individuals, families and communities to promote independence, provide support and prevent harm, neglect and abuse.

- **Contexts and organisations**

  Engage with, inform, and adapt to changing contexts that shape practice. Operate effectively within your own organisational frameworks and contribute to the development of services and organisations. Operate effectively within multi-agency and inter-professional settings.

- **Professional leadership**

  Take responsibility for the professional learning and development of others through supervision, mentoring, assessing, research, teaching, leadership and management.

  References to these standards will be made throughout the text and you will find a diagram of the Professional Capability Framework in Appendix 1 on page 220.

This book will help students to meet the demands outlined by the Department of Health in the prescribed curriculum and especially in relation to the expressed need that all social workers must understand about mental health and how to work with colleagues from other disciplines.

This book will help students to meet the social work subject benchmarks published in April 2008 by the Quality Assurance Agency for Higher Education. These are incorporated at the start of each chapter. These include being able to understand the nature of social work and developing knowledge and understanding about the following:

- social work services and service users;
- values and ethics;
- social work theory; and
- the nature of social work practice.

Book structure

Mental health services seem to be in a state of continual change. The latest policy **No Health Without Mental Health** (2012) brings together much of the last decade's previous ideas and the Equality Act 2010 provides important protection for people including people with mental health problems. After a long wait the 2007 Mental Health Act was a major and substantial amendment to the 1983 Mental Health Act. With the accompanying changes to the Mental Capacity Act and the two new Codes of Practice the next few years will be both interesting and challenging. Meanwhile new government policies have come into being that will provide welcome boosts to funding for dementia, surely one of the great challenges facing society. Although integrated services are high on this agenda it remains my view that social work should be at the heart of these changes and a crucial part of delivering improved services for vulnerable people. This book has in its own modest way a part to play in the transformation of future social work practice.

The beginning of the book has a clear focus upon values and the importance of social workers underpinning their practice with values and principles that demonstrate that they can work with diverse populations, some of whom experience disadvantage and oppression. The examples of work with black and minority ethnic communities and people who are deaf, serve to demonstrate the necessity for culturally sensitive practice.

In Chapter 2 the medical model is described in detail, as this remains the dominant approach to work with service users. However, it is not the only approach and the case is put that a more socially oriented approach needs to be understood by social workers as well as the medical approach. This orientation is about more than providing services to support medical interventions: it takes into account a more holistic view of the confusing and contradictory world of mental disorder. To help understand this, emphasis is placed on the role that stress has as an intervening variable that increases the vulnerability of people to mental disorder. Such stressful events can include life events or circumstances such as unemployment or relationship breakdown.

The law is never far from mental health social work and Chapter 3 examines the legal and political context in which social workers, approved social workers and the approved mental health worker will find themselves. The case for and against compulsory admission is made and the process covered. Emphasis is placed on human rights and how they are incorporated into the legislation, and how the various community care initiatives can allow imaginative solutions for helping people return to or remain in the community. The main provisions refer only to the law in England.

Chapter 4 covers Mental Health Tribunals and looks in detail at the role of social workers in preparing and delivering Social Circumstance Reports. Later in the chapter mental capacity and important concepts such as Deprivation of Liberty Safeguards are covered in detail. As an extreme example, the publicly held tribunal of the 'moors murderer' Ian Brady is discussed as it raises interesting issues.

Chapter 5 examines work with children and adolescents and the range of interventions in this area of work. The Child and Adolescent Mental Health Service, although slow to get underway, is for the foreseeable future what services will look like despite funding cuts. The example of eating disorder is covered in some detail to provide an example of work with adolescents. LGBT issues are covered and used an example of best practice.

Working with service users who are short-term users of mental health services provides the content of Chapter 6. In particular, the task facing social workers who are working with people who are at risk of suicide provides the subject matter, with an illustrative example that runs throughout most of the chapter. The importance of understanding the research evidence that frames our work in any area is given emphasis.

Chapter 7 looks at work with service users who have long-term or chronic needs. The illustrative example of a man diagnosed with schizophrenia is used and in particular the concept of early intervention and family work are suggested as ways that effective intervention can be accomplished. Stressful situations can include families that have 'high expressed emotion' and this is used to demonstrate effective work with families. The differences in diagnosis between African-Caribbean young men and their white counterparts are explored, and the concept of risk is briefly examined.

The final chapter returns the reader to work with children and the concept of working across professional and organisational boundaries. This covers the importance of child protection and the case of Victoria Climbié. Learning lessons from Inquiries includes learning how to work better together – the Allitt Inquiry raises important issues of which social work professionals should be aware. Children whose parents separate can respond adversely to the stresses that this event can create. Yet others get by and even thrive in later life, and their resilience and ability to bounce back is considered in detail as it provides an important series of pointers as to where intervention could be targeted.

Finally some signposts for the future are aired during the last few pages.

Learning features

As far as a book can be, this has been written to help you to interact with the material as an active participant. The combination of this book, liberal use of the internet and self-reflection should ensure effective learning.

Case studies are used throughout the book to help make real the application of the theory to practice. To add interest some historical notes are provided, especially in Chapter 3.

We know that approximately one in six people in England experience mental health problems at any given time and that some groups of people are more susceptible than others. Social work students and social workers are no different and it is important that this book recognises this and in a small way provides not just intellectual rigour but practical advice. Throughout this book stress is seen as something that can tip someone from being mentally healthy into having a mental health problem. This can be a single event although often it is a build-up of little things. These need to be dealt with and some chapters provide tips to bust your stress.

There is a 'companion' text in this series that you may want to consult by John Archambeault (2009) *Social Work and Mental Health* as well as the excellent Martin Webber (2011) *Evidence-based Policy and Practice in Mental Health.*

Chapter 1

Values and ethical mental health social work

ACHIEVING A SOCIAL WORK DEGREE

This chapter will help you to develop the following capabilities from the **Professional Capabilities Framework**:

- **Professionalism**
  Identify and behave as a professional social worker committed to professional development.

- **Values and ethics**
  Apply social work ethical principles and values to guide professional practice.

- **Knowledge**
  Apply knowledge of social sciences, law and social work practice theory.

- **Critical reflection and analysis**
  Apply critical reflection and analysis to inform and provide a rationale for professional decision-making.

- **Intervention and skills**
  Use judgement and authority to intervene with individuals, families and communities to promote independence, provide support and prevent harm, neglect and abuse.

It will also introduce you to the following standards as set out in the 2008 social work subject benchmark statement:

5.1.3   Values and ethics.
5.1.5   The nature of social work practice.

Introduction

The World Heath Organisation describes **mental health** as:

> a state of well-being in which the individual realizes his or her abilities, can cope with the normal stresses of life, can work productively and fruitfully, and is able to make a contribution to his or her community.
>
> MENTAL ill health includes mental health problems and strain; impaired functioning associated with distress, symptoms, and diagnosable mental health disorders, such as schizophrenia and depression.

> *The mental condition of people is determined by a multiplicity of factors including biological, individual, family and social, economic and environmental.*
>
> (European Commission Green Paper, 2005, p.4)

This chapter examines the relationship between values, ethics, contemporary social work and social care practice in the Mental Health Services. Mental health services are at a crucial stage of redevelopment which, by the time it is complete, will produce a service that is appropriate and responsive to service user needs. Values and ethics are at the heart of culturally competent professional practice. This means that social workers will be able to value their own culture and be able to work in a sensitive manner with people from other cultures. To become culturally competent requires empathy, understanding and acceptance of differences (Walker, 2003; see also culturally sensitive practice in *Engaging and Changing*, Patel, 2003).

Approximately one person in six, at some time in their life, will experience mental health problems that are sufficiently serious for them to seek help from a professional. It is usually the family doctor who is the first port of call and they in turn refer people on to the various agencies whose remit is to provide mental health services. These services include health, social care and social work agencies that are trying to work together to provide a seamless service for the user. Some GP practices have social workers attached to them and this often means that these workers will be doing direct work with service users, working in the community alongside other mental health professionals, or be working in a psychiatric hospital. Social workers also come across mental health problems in addition to the 'presenting problem' that led to referral in the first place.

Basic facts

The following are extracted from the current mental health policy **No Health Without Mental Health** (2011).

- At least one in four people will experience mental health problems at some point in their lives and one in six has a problem at any one time.

- One in ten children between 5 and 16 years have a mental health problem and many will continue throughout their adult live to have similar problems.

- Half of those with lifetime mental health problems experienced symptoms by the age of 14¾ before their mid-20s.

- 10–13% of 15–16 year olds have self-harmed.

- Almost half of all adults will experience at least one episode of depression during their lifetime.

- One in ten new mothers have experienced post-natal depression.

- About one in 100 people have a severe mental health problem.

- 60% of people living in hostels have a personality disorder.

- Some 90% of all prisoners are estimated to have a diagnosable mental health problem or a substance misuse problem.

Of course you need to treat all such statistics with caution but even if there are some discrepancies with the above they still show mental health to be one of the most pressing of issues that we as a society are facing and you and me as social workers are working with.

A strategy for the mental health of the European Union

In January 2005 the World Health Organisation held a conference for European Ministers to start a process of drawing up a framework for comprehensive action and political commitment for mental health. The subsequent Green Paper is an important contribution to setting up a series of actions that may prove to be a significant initiative. The purpose was to stimulate debate within Europe and to engage a broad range of institutions, health professionals, social care professionals, research communities and service users, in discussions about how best to improve public mental health.

Three areas for improvement are identified:

Mental ill health affects every fourth citizen and can lead to suicide, a cause of too many deaths.

Mental ill health causes significant losses and burdens to the economic, social, educational as well as criminal and justice systems.

Stigmatisation, discrimination and non-respect for the human rights and the dignity of mentally ill and disabled people still exist, challenging core European values.

(European Commission Green Paper, 2005)

The Paper goes on to describe how mental health is a growing challenge to the EU and to support the WHO view that by 2020 depression will be the highest ranking cause of disease in the developed world (WHO, 2001). Other statistics include the statement that:

Currently, in the EU, some 58,000 citizens die from suicide every year, more than from the annual deaths from road accidents, homicide or HIV/AIDS.

(Green Paper, p.4)

Clearly there are significant inequalities within member states and this reflects the richness and diverse nature of the EU but nevertheless the Paper proposes that a strategy would be focused upon prevention of mental ill health, the improvement of the quality of life for people with mental health and the development of a mental health information and research system for the EU.

Mental health strategy in the UK

Each country in the United Kingdom has developed policies with social inclusion as a major issue. With the exception of Northern Ireland these have been developed in the period 2012/13 and are summarised below.

The strategy for England

The government has set about improving mental health care in general. Key policy documents are **No Health Without Mental Health; A cross-government mental health outcomes strategy for people of all ages** (February 2011) and **No Health Without Mental Health: Implementation Strategy** (24 July 2012). The Health and Social Care Act 2012 makes it explicit that mental health problems should be treated the same as physical health problems. This framework for 2012/1013 has three improvement areas:

- Reduction of early deaths among people with serious mental illness.
- Improving employment prospects for people with mental illness.
- Improve patient experience of community mental health teams.

One of the key tasks for the reformed services is to combat the effects of social exclusion and to provide a service that is user-focused. The idea is that through a combination of policy initiatives people will feel that they have a greater sense of belonging to a community and services will form new partnerships between the providers and recipients of services. Thus various initiatives have been put in place to meet the needs of specific populations such as women, people who are deaf, and black and minority ethnic groups.

This more inclusive approach has a focus on community-based services, which has been a trend over the last two decades, but the new strategy takes this further with local commissioning of services and a focus upon outcome evaluation against various targets. As this focus upon local services continues, the danger is that services will become more fragmented. With decentralised structures there is a need to establish general standards against which these communities' services can be judged and these are already in place.

These standards need to be seen alongside the more specific inspection standards for the Care Quality Commission, which in 2009 replaced the Healthcare Commission (which replaced the Commission for Social Care Inspection (CSCI), the successor in April 2004 to the National Care Standards Commission (NCSC)). After considerable public disquiet about the performance of the CQC in July 2013 it remains to be seen if they too are to be replaced!

Meeting tough outcomes is a challenge to agencies as well as to individual practitioners. As a social worker you may be working with service users and communities as well as other professionals to plan, implement and evaluate mental health services. The emphases on user empowerment, community development and non-discriminatory services are all part of the tool kit that you, as a social worker, will be expected to develop.

Before you can begin to consider yourself an effective mental health social worker you need to understand the values that underpin professional practice and how they are reflected in agency policy and practice and endorsed in governmental policies. You need to understand the part that you will play as a social worker/social care worker in the modernising agenda. It is important that as a developing professional your practice demonstrates commitment to promoting equality. Regardless of the language of different policies the aim is to modernise services and to promote the integration of health and social care services within mental health trusts so that they provide a seamless provision for service users though this may be at a price to the profession of social work. *The emphasis on professional collaboration and integration has sparked concerns that the distinctive contribution of social work in mental health services might be diminished* (SCIE Research briefing 26, 2008).

The strategy for Wales

Similar to the strategy for England but adjusted to better meet the needs of the Welsh people is **Together for Health**, the Welsh government's five-year vision for the NHS that good health is vital to the creation of a prosperous, successful and sustainable Wales. Addressing the disadvantages faced by people with mental illness and ensuring equal access to care and treatment is essential to this. **Together for Mental Health** builds on developments in mental health services over the last 10 years, including the legal requirements of **The Mental Health (Wales) Measure 2010**. It takes this work forward, providing a long-term commitment to improve mental health and wellbeing backed by significant funding.

At its heart the Strategy is to improve mental health among the population and to improve services for people of all ages including children and young people. Central to this approach is the idea of recovery and the route to this will be through more effective partnerships both with the general population and through an effective network of services.

The Welsh Strategy has six high level outcomes:

- The mental health and wellbeing of the whole population is improved.

- The impact of mental health problems and/or mental illness on individuals of all ages, their families and carers, communities and the economy more widely, is better recognised and reduced.

- Inequalities, stigma and discrimination suffered by people experiencing mental health problems and mental illness are reduced.

- Individuals have a better experience of the support and treatment they receive and have an increased feeling of input and control over related decisions.

- Access to, and the quality of preventative measures, early intervention and treatment services are improved and more people recover as a result.

- The values, attitudes and skills of those treating or supporting individuals of all ages with mental health problems or mental illness are improved.

(Welsh Government, 2012, p.7)

5

Want to read more then access:

http://wales.gov.uk/docs/dhss/publications/130328mhsummaryen.pdf

For the 10-year strategy:

http://wales.gov.uk/docs/dhss/publications/121031tmhfinalen.pdf

The strategy for Scotland

In Scotland the **Mental Health Strategy 2012–15**, launched in August 2012, and sharing many of the characteristics of the other countries, supports and adopts the three Quality Ambitions for Scotland that health and care is person centred, safe and effective. There are seven key themes and 36 specific commitments to be delivered over the period to 2015 and these cover the full spectrum of mental health improvement, prevention, care, services, and recovery.

The seven key themes:

- Working more effectively with families and carers.

- Embedding more peer to peer work and support.

- Increasing the support for self-management and self-help approaches.

- Extending the anti-stigma agenda forward to include further work on discrimination.

- Focusing on the rights of those with mental illness.

- Developing the outcomes approach to include personal, social and clinical outcomes.

- Ensuring that we use new technology effectively as a mechanism for providing information and delivering evidence based services.

(August 2012, Scottish Government)

The Mental Health Strategy includes:

- promoting good mental health;

- improving access to psychological therapies;

- better access to Child and Adolescent Mental Health Services;

- reducing stigma and discrimination for people with mental health problems;

- rights and recovery and employability;

- removing unnecessary barriers between services.

Want to read more then access:

www.scotland.gov.uk/Topics/Health/Services/Mental-Health/Strategy

The strategy for Northern Ireland

In Northern Ireland the strategy goes back to 2009 when the NI Executive envisaged a 15-year plan to improve mental health and services for people with mental health problems. This cross-departmental Action Plan sets out the key actions that will be taken forward in response to the 'Bamford Review' recommendations. The main aim is to protect and preserve the mental health of the population as a whole, where possible to promote better mental health for everyone and to improve the lives of those with a learning disability or a mental health need.

> To make the Bamford vision a reality, the NI Executive will promote the mental wellbeing of the population as a whole. The Executive will also promote the health and wellbeing, and maximise the independence and full participation of people of all ages with a mental health need or a learning disability, underpinned by legislation and public services to include reform and modernisation of mental health and learning disability services. People with a mental health need or a learning disability using public services should expect to:
>
> be encouraged and supported to look after their own health, both mental and physical, and build up emotional resilience;
>
> be supported, as far as possible, in their own homes and communities, making best use of self-directed help; be supported, through effective collaboration between Government Departments and their agencies, in their life choices and in day to day activities of engaging in education, training, work and leisure;
>
> be consulted on and be able to influence the provision of services to meet their needs;
>
> be encouraged to access help at as early a stage as possible; and
>
> be supported towards personal fulfillment and full citizenship.
>
> (Department of Health, Social Services and Public Safety, 2012)

Why not read *Delivering the Bamford Vision: the response of NI Executive to the Bamford review of mental health and learning disability. Action Plan 2009-2011.*

Access at: **www.dhsspsni.gov.uk/bamford_action_plan_2009-2011.pdf**

Unpicking the policy for England

Present-day life in government departments must be a dizzying experience as staff try to produce or perhaps even keep abreast of new initiatives. To do so is very important for social workers and as a student you need to develop the habit of reading and critically appraising policy documents and legislation. This is the case even if at first glance such initiatives seem not to be directly related to your area of practice. I have singled out two key papers to help provide the context in which you as a social worker will practise. These are referred to later on in the book but here is a brief summary of the key points.

No Health Without Mental Health

Policy surrounding mental health has been hurtling its way around the web over the last decade and not always with the effect that was intended. The most recent policy **No Health Without Mental Health** was launched by Deputy Prime Minister Nick Clegg in 2011. The strategy is worth reading and reflecting on as it represents a change in government thinking. The underlying rationale for this is that if mental health and wellbeing is to be promoted and improved then this can only be done at the local level. This marks a significant change and affects the way in services are commissioned, designed and delivered. This in turn has resulted in new structures that will enable local providers, with the support of government, to translate policy into practice with a degree of local flavour. In the foreword to the strategy Sir David Nicholson, NHS Chief Executive, NHS Commissioning Board and Duncan Selbie, Chief Executive Designate Public Health England wrote:

> *The reform of the health and care system provides a significant opportunity to improve people's mental health and wellbeing. It is an opportunity we are determined to take as the new organisations and systems take shape.*
>
> *We are committed to improving the mental health and wellbeing of the whole population, and the life chances of people with mental health conditions. We are determined to ensure mental health has equal priority with physical health, a principle enshrined in the Health and Social Care Act 2012.*
>
> *As the NHS Commissioning Board and Public Health England come into being, we will ensure that improving mental health and wellbeing is integral to all of the key functions and approaches in both organisations, and that we provide clear leadership in ensuring equal priority for mental health.*
>
> *The implementation challenge and the actions suggested in this framework now need to be taken up fully and enthusiastically across the NHS, the new public health system, and the public, private and voluntary organisations that all have a unique role to play in improving people's mental health.*
>
> (DoH, 2012)

This strategy sits in among a tidal wave of other related policies including the NHS White Paper *Equality and Excellence: Liberating the NHS and Healthy Lives, Healthy People: the strategy for public health in England*.

All government policies look good, but then much of government policy often does, but fine words do not make fine services and it is to the *implementation framework* that our hopes must rest. This document sets out just how some of this, it has to be said, ambitious policy to put mental health on a par with physical health by the direct provision of services and ideas to tackle attitudes to mental health in local services, businesses and communities. Included in these initiatives is the plan to Improving Access to Psychological Therapies (IAPT) with overall estimates of cost set at £400 million which is thought to be an effective way of responding to mental health issues. This framework complements other governmental programmes in 2014 including the **Prime Minister's Challenge on Dementia** and the programme for **support for women with postnatal depression**.

The framework has been produced by the Department of Health with five leading mental health organisations: Centre for Mental Health; Mind; NHS Confederation Mental Health Network; Rethink Mental Illness; and Turning Point. Like all of these documents it is readily available on the web and in a range of formats. They are worth visiting as this framework highlights useful guidance and sources of information to help local organisations use their existing powers and resources to improve mental health and wellbeing.

The framework has six areas within which outcomes will be determined:

1. More people have better mental health – more people of all ages and backgrounds will have better wellbeing and good mental health.

2. More people recover from mental illness – this includes a better quality of life and improved chances in education and employment.

3. People with mental illness have better physical health – the aim is to reduce the number of premature deaths among people with mental health problems and improve the mental health of those with physical health problems.

4. Positive experience of care and support – care and support should be timely and effective with choice of treatment available to people.

5. Fewer people suffer avoidable harm – increase the confidence level of people who use mental health services.

6. Fewer people experience stigma and discrimination – improve the public awareness and understanding of mental health

These are all interconnected and some more than others. I have set aside two areas with obvious connections and these are in Figure 1.1.

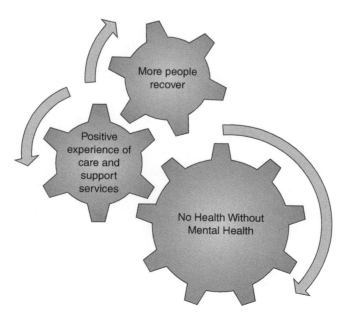

Figure 1.1   Example of connectedness of outcomes to policy

How are these outcomes to be measured? If we take the example above and break each of the cogs into specific outcomes then the following emerges – 'More people recover' measured by:

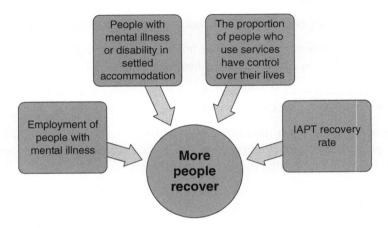

Figure 1.2   'More people recover'

The same process applied to 'Positive experience of care and support services' reveals outcomes as follows:

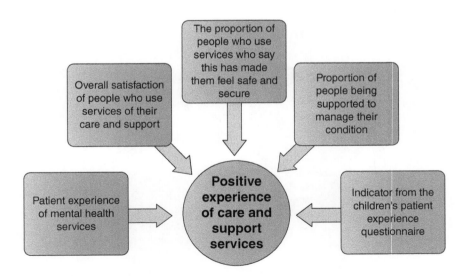

Figure 1.3   Positive outcomes of services

The importance of values

Social work is fundamentally a moral activity. Social workers often refer to values; indeed Clark (2000) suggests that values are the staple diet of social workers although the word is used indiscriminately when principles or ethics would be more accurate. Clark suggests that there are four core values:

1. The worth and uniqueness of each individual.

2. The entitlement to justice.

3. The essentiality of community.

4. The claim to freedom.

These values were given statutory force through the National Health Service and Community Care Act (DoH, 1990) and various practice guidance notes including *Valuing People* (DoH, 2001) that stress not only the importance of these values but require services and practitioners to uphold them.

Values, knowledge and skills are interconnected in everyday practice even though this is not always apparent. Figure 1.4 shows how these are connected to each other.

Since April 2005 the title of social worker become legally protected and hence only those who are registered can call themselves social workers. The Health Care Professions Council (HCPC), which took over as the regulatory body in 2012, declare that they will prosecute anyone who makes a false claim to be a social worker. The Register also permits easy confirmation that someone is currently registered and not subject to disciplinary matters. In addition to the Code of Practice the HCPC, along with the College of Social Work, has set out a Professional Capabilities

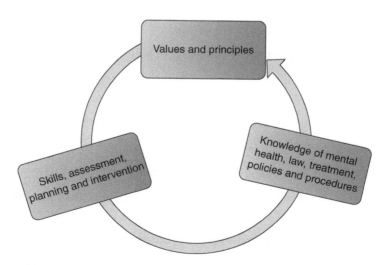

Figure 1.4   Values, knowledge and skills: the foundations of good practice

Framework that sets out what you need to achieve in order to be awarded a social work degree. The overall aim is to drive up the standards of social work and those who practise as social workers (See Appendix 1, p. 220). Values of course underpin practice, and the relationship to skills and knowledge are illustrated in Figure 1.4.

You might at this point be asking why do we need a Code of Professional Practice and this becomes apparent when you begin to learn about the role that social workers have alongside other professionals who deliver mental health services. At times, people with mental health problems can be in such a vulnerable state that they may even require admission to hospital against their wishes. They need to be assured that nationally agreed standards of service delivery are being adhered to and that the service provider can be held accountable when services fall short. Different professions have their own codes of practice and conduct, which have three common themes:

- the avoidance of possible harm to services users;
- the promotion of possible good to service users;
- the protection of the profession and the resolution of conflicts.

Code of Practice

The HCPC has published a Code of Practice that sets out the standards of conduct, performance and ethics that are expected of you as a student and later as a qualified registered social worker. Although students are not registered you will need to apply for registration once qualified and in order for you to correctly call yourself a social worker. This acts as a framework in which you practise and in my opinion you should work within this irrespective of your status. Having read this you could be forgiven for thinking that practice is like walking on eggshells but in reality the essence of your practice should be to make informed, reasonable and professional judgements in a rational manner (with your service users as your prime concern) that enables you to justify any decisions if you are asked to do so.

1. **You should always act in the best interests of your service users.**

   - You should respect a person's right to have their interventions carried out by a professional and not a student.
   - You should not exploit or abuse your relationships with service users.
   - You should treat everyone equally.
   - You should not do anything that you think will put someone in danger.
   - If you are worried about a situation, which might put someone at risk, you should speak to a member of the placement team or your education provider.

2. **You should respect the confidentiality of your service users.**

   - You should keep information about service users confidential, and only use it for the purpose for which it was given, unless the information raises concerns about a situation where someone may be at risk.

- You should not knowingly give any personal or confidential information to anyone who is not entitled to access it.

- You should remove anything that could be used to identify a service user from confidential information, which you use in your assessment.

- You should follow local policies or guidelines if you want to use information that may identify someone in your assessments.

- You should follow local policies or guidelines on confidentiality produced by your education provider or placement provider.

3. You should keep high standards of personal conduct.

You should be aware that conduct outside of your programme might affect whether or not you are allowed to complete your programme or register with us.

Guidance on conduct and ethics for students

- You should be polite with service users, your colleagues and the programme team.

- You should make sure that your personal appearance is appropriate for your placement environment.

- You should follow your education provider's or placement provider's policy on attendance.

4. You should provide any important information about your conduct, competence or health to your education provider.

- You should tell your education provider and placement provider about any existing health conditions or changes to your health, which may put your service users or yourself at risk.

- You should tell your education provider if you are convicted of, or cautioned for, any offence.

5. You should limit your study or stop studying if your performance or judgement is affected by your health.

- You should get help from a doctor or an occupational health professional if you are worried about your health.

- You should be aware that you might put your service users or yourself at risk if your performance or judgement is affected by your health.

6. You should keep your professional knowledge and skills up to date.

- You are responsible for your own learning.

- You should think about and respond positively to feedback you are given.

7. You should act within the limits of your knowledge and skills.

You should only carry out an unsupervised task if you feel that you have the appropriate knowledge and skills.

8. **You should communicate effectively with service users and your education provider and placement providers.**

   - You should take all reasonable steps to make sure that you can communicate appropriately and effectively with service users.

   - You should communicate effectively and cooperate with colleagues to benefit service users.

   - You should communicate effectively and cooperate with the programme team and placement team.

   - Where appropriate, you should share your knowledge with colleagues.

9. **You should get informed consent to provide care or services (so far as possible).**

   Informed consent is when someone has all the information they need, in a format they can understand, to make a decision about receiving care or services.

   You should do the following (so far as possible).

   - You should make sure that before you carry out any intervention, the service user is aware that you are a student.

   - You should make sure that the service user has given their permission for the intervention to be carried out by a student.

   - You should explain the intervention you are planning to carry out.

   - Before you carry out any intervention, you should explain any risks associated with it.

   - You should follow your education provider's or placement provider's policy on consent.

10. **You should keep accurate records on service users.**

    - You should make sure that any information you put in someone's record is accurate and clear.

    - You should protect information in records from being lost, damaged, accessed by someone without permission or tampered with.

11. **You should deal fairly and safely with the risks of infection.**

    - You should make sure that you take all appropriate steps to deal with the risks of infection.

    - You should follow your education provider's or placement provider's policy on managing the risks of infection.

12. **You should behave honestly.**

    - You should not pass off other people's work as your own.

    - You should make sure that you reference other people's work appropriately.

    - You should make sure that you truthfully and accurately fill in any documents.

- You should not let any improper financial reward influence the advice and services you provide, or the products you recommend.

- You should follow your education provider's policies on ethics when carrying out research.

13. **You should make sure that your behaviour does not damage public confidence in your profession.**

- You should be aware that your behaviour might affect the trust that the public has in your profession.

- You should not do anything which might affect the trust that the public has in your profession.

As a student you should also consider the following:

Guidance on conduct and ethics for students

- You should make sure that you are appropriately supervised for any task that you are asked to carry out.

- You should ask for help when you need it.

- You should make sure that you do not claim that you have knowledge and skills, which you do not.

The full document from which the above is derived can be accessed from: **www.hpc-uk.org/publications/**

How are you going to be guided by values and ethics?

ACTIVITY *1.1*

Look at your Code of Practice, the basics of which are set out above. Taking all the aspects reorder them to fit into the framework proposed earlier:

- ones that avoid possible harm to service users;

- ones that promote possible good to service users;

- ones that protect the profession and resolve conflicts.

What is the balance between these? To what extent are these about risk management?

Values in action

Implicit in the Code of Professional Social Work Practice is the importance of recognising and respecting diversity. This is more than valuing people irrespective of their race, colour or ability. It also involves valuing and respecting that people think and behave differently. People of all ethnic backgrounds and countries experience mental disorder and the service user population is made up of people just like you and me.

Conventionally and stereotypically medical practice has remained the dominant partner through its claim to be a series of technical activities that can be evidenced by rigorous research. Advances in medication have reinforced the idea that an individual's mental disorder can be managed and that the key process is diagnosis followed by treatment monitoring and evaluation. In this process the danger is that the treated are subservient to those in charge of treatment.

Social workers need to work with medical and health colleagues to provide an effective service but they also need to be at the forefront of processes that empower service users. Implicit in this approach are some ordinary but powerful principles.

The first is that in order to empower someone we need to work with them rather than do things to them. Empowerment means partnership, openness and honesty.

The second principle is that the service user has an explanation of their disorder. That needs understanding and to achieve this we need to find ways of active listening that respect the user and enable us to do our job. This may mean having to use imaginative ways of communicating. It might mean trying to use a common language, which could be sign language. It should mean engaging in clear, uncomplicated language that everyone can understand.

The third principle is that service users value being able to engage with professionals on a personal level. This could mean that social workers should learn to use 'limited' self-disclosure to help build up professional relationships that are also person-to-person, not expert to amateur (Blackburn and Golightley, 2004). Being able to walk in the other person's shoes is an important part of an empowering approach.

The fourth principle is that the service user is the expert in their own mental health problem. They may not know the answers but they certainly experience the effect or symptoms. They alone have experienced the disintegration of 'normality' as they know it and their explanation should be put alongside the professional view and the two views evaluated against each other. If your world is upside down or inside out it cannot be understood by people who only see things one way up or right side out. If a service user is hearing voices the social worker must not dismiss these but try to understand when they arrive, what they feel like and how best they can be managed. This is not to collude with delusional behaviour as this could be unhelpful and possibly run the risk of missing dangerous behaviour.

By working with service users to value their experiences, and by seeing the problem through their eyes, the prospect is opened up to work in a manner that is holistic and empowering.

The significance of social work perspectives and values

In a very interesting publication by SCIE (research briefing 26 July 2008) research has been drawn together to show the value that service users place on non-stigmatising help and access to services that are provided by social workers. They write:

Similarly, analysis of the 'essential capabilities' required to practice in mental health also emphasises the importance of a professional value base which promotes dignity, human worth and social justice ... indeed, research exploring community care practices found that social workers frequently identified empowerment as a fundamental principle in their practice, both as a goal and as an underpinning value.

(SCIE no 26, p.4)

This is such a clear statement that sums up a perspective that is unique to social work and when put alongside an understanding of the impact of social exclusion and social injustice and oppression puts social workers in a good position to be able to work positively with people who are susceptible to discriminatory practices including lesbian, gay and transgender and black and minority ethnic communities.

Ethical dilemmas

Health and social care workers face dilemmas on a daily basis. There are usually two components that help us to think about ethical dilemmas. First there may be competing views about what should be done. How would you respond to a service user when they want to stop taking their medicine? This is an ethical dilemma and people would argue strongly for one position or the other. This contrasts with a view that medicine should be given with or without service user consent, if it were necessary to prevent death or serious harm occurring. In this instance this is not an ethical issue as there is widespread agreement. (Even so some people claim this should not happen, usually on religious grounds.)

The second characteristic is that it must have a distinct moral component to it, such as the avoidance of lying, the primacy of life, self-determination and confidentiality. These characteristics are sometimes referred to as 'normative principles'.

Resolving ethical dilemmas takes more than just referring to these normative principles or the various codes of conduct. It requires professional judgements after weighing up one principle against another. The following activity will help you to think further about the ethical dilemmas.

ACTIVITY **1.2**

Sanjay is a long-term service user who has recurring bouts of depression, which are serious enough to warrant his treatment with anti-depressants. In the past when his mood has been very low he has talked about 'ending it all'. As his social worker you visit regularly and he tells you in confidence that he has stopped his medicati experiment with herbal medicine, which is more usual in his culture. opinion about this action and told you to keep this conversation confi respect his wishes? Jot down what your response would be and what compare with the following paragraphs.

18

(Continued)

COMMENT

If anyone wants to stop taking medication then this is their right under common law. In certain circumstances, and providing that they are detained under the Mental Health Act 1983, they can be made to have treatment against their wishes. Sanjay can stop his medication although whether this is a good thing is open to debate.

Arguments against keeping confidences or keeping matters confidential derive from different sources. First there is a principle of paternalism usually derived from the possession of 'expert' knowledge. Put crudely the professional knows best. Second there is a principle of autonomy where the person has freedom over their own body, which is essentially a moral principle. Individuals are experts in their own mental health condition and as such they know best. Resolution of this requires you to balance the strength of one principle against the other. In practice you would probably seek to encourage Sanjay to sit with the others involved in his treatment and to talk through his and your concerns and try to get to a position where his shift to herbal remedies is informed by evidence, monitored and reviewed.

You would need to take into account the extent to which the service user has the capacity to be able to make such a decision, the quality of the information on which this is based, if there was any coercion on the service user when making this decision and any legal issues that could change the nature of the discussion.

One way that service users can be helped to make good quality decisions is through patient advocacy services. By using advocates who are independent of the mental health team, but who have specific knowledge of mental health and mental health services, the quality of service user decisions can be enhanced.

Ethnicity and mental health

The discrimination that is experienced by people with mental health problems can be intensified if that person happens to be from a black and minority ethnic community. A service user talks about her experience of using mental health services as a black person:

> *Coming to mental health services was like the last straw ... you come to services disempowered already, they strip you of your dignity ... you become the dregs of society.*

(Keating and Robertson, 2002, p.18)

This is a commonly held experience of black service users. When put together with the perception that when black people are seen as difficult they are likely to be over medicated there is little wonder that this has become a priority area.

Discrimination has been a source of concern to many practitioners over the years. Evidence has suggested that on the one hand the UK's black and minority ethnic population are over-represented in secondary care (hospital admissions, etc.) and on the other hand under-represented in primary care that specifically addresses the needs of black and minority ethnic communities. Of particular concern has been the over-representation of African-Caribbean people who have been detained against their will and who are being treated in Medium Secure Hospitals (MSUs). Evidence collected by the Mental Health Act Commission shows that 30% of the population resident in MSUs were from predominantly African-Caribbean ethnic groups, which is well over the proportion that might be expected when compared with the population at large. African-Caribbean people living in the UK have lower rates of common mental disorders than other ethnic groups but are more likely to be diagnosed with severe mental illness. African-Caribbean people are three to five times more likely than any other group to be diagnosed and admitted to hospital for schizophrenia (Mental Health Foundation).

Fundamental to developing better social work practice is having better quality of information and using it more intelligently than is evident at present. A starting point is for you to become familiar with population data and information about ethnic minorities.

ACTIVITY 1.3

The proportion of black and minority ethnic groups in the UK rose from 6% to 9% over the period 1991–2001. The African-Caribbean population in England and Wales is about 2%. This does vary considerably depending on where you live and work. Commonly members of the public at large over-estimate the numbers of black and minority ethnic populations. Think about why this is, what influences this perception and what some of the implications of this might be. Write down why you think some ethnic groups are thought to be larger than they actually, are, what influences this perception and some of the implications of this.

COMMENT

You probably came up with the idea that the media plays a big role here with some of the less sophisticated newspapers in particular promoting the idea that we are being over-populated with asylum seekers, drug users and the like. Mental health is not the only area where we see statistics that ought to concern us: the Sunday Times *(14 December 2003) reported, 'twice as many black people are in prison as at university'. They report that the Race Relations watchdog has concluded that while 10,000 African-Caribbean people are in jails – a much higher percentage than to be expected – the numbers at university are only about 5,000.*

Providing mental health services that are, and need to be seen to be, responsive to the needs of individuals requires that they should reflect the rich diversity that makes up our society. However, in the late 1980s it was becoming apparent that although moves were being made to promote patient-centred services, this did nothing to address the specific needs of the black and minority ethnic communities.

Although these views were commonly held throughout health and social care, social work was one of the few professions that placed special emphasis on training in anti-racist and anti-discriminatory practice. At the policy level, the government's Modernisation Plan and the Mental Health National Service Framework (1999) sets out in Standard One the need to combat discrimination against individuals and groups with mental health problems and promote their social inclusion. This has built on the legal foundation laid down in the Human Rights Act 1998, the introduction of the Race Relations (Amendment) Act 2000 and the Equality Act 2010.

More recently the Department of Health embarked on an impressive and ambitious change agenda called *Delivering Race Equality: A Framework for Action* (October 2003). Although this programme formally came to a conclusion in March 2010 many areas have continued the work and you can see one example in the east Midlands by accessing **www.eastmids.org.uk**. It is disappointing that just as this programme was getting underway it was stopped and much remains to be done. However there are valuable lessons that we have learnt and in the foreword to the evaluation of the programme Luis Appleby wrote:

> DRE's work has informed New Horizons: towards a shared vision for mental health, our new vision for mental health in England, which builds on the 1999 National Service Framework for Mental Health (NSF). New Horizons and its associated equality impact assessment described the evidence for the – often very serious – inequalities in mental health among some ethnic groups. The roots of these inequalities lay in social, not biological, factors so the responsibility for remedial action extends to all the agencies that influence public mental health and well-being.
>
> (DoH, 2009)

The present approach falls out of the Health and Social Care Act 2012 where the concentration now comes under the umbrella term 'reducing inequalities in health' and further information is provided through some helpful 'fact sheets' – this particular one is Factsheet C2 which provides details regarding health inequalities and the Health and Social Care Act 2012. It is part of a wide range of factsheets on the Act, all available at: **www.dh.gov.uk/healthandsocialcarebill**

What does this mean for mental health social work practice?

James Nazroo (1999) suggests that different rates of diagnosis of mental illness between black and minority ethnic people represent one of the most controversial issues that present-day services face. In practical terms you need to examine the reasons why minority groups such as African-Caribbean men are six times more likely to be compulsorily detained than white people, why Asian women are more likely to be depressed than their white counterparts and why minority ethnic groups are less likely to seek early help from primary care.

Mental health is a significant area of social work practice, which will bring you face to face with people who may be vulnerable and confused. As a social worker you need to work together with other professionals in a way that is person-centered and upholds human rights. This is far from straightforward, with tension and conflict possible at virtually every stage of your work. Such tension can exist between for example:

- the wishes of the service user and their families;

- the need to protect the public and the need to promote service user independence;

- and, as you saw earlier, the right to refuse treatment and the need to have treatment.

In trying to work with these tensions you will often find yourself playing a crucial role in any decision-making context.

Anti-oppressive practice

Social work has a history of attempts to practise in ways that are anti-oppressive. One of the key figures in the literature is Dominelli whose book *Anti-Racist Social Work* (1988) not only provides well-argued discussion about these issues but also gives strategies for the implementation of anti-racist social work. These ideas, although over two decades old, still have relevance for you as a practitioner as mental health care is the only aspect of care provision and treatment that, if refused, can result in that person's compulsory admission to hospital through a legally authorised pathway. Indeed recent research suggests that service users value the non-stigmatising help and access to services that social workers provide and that these are entirely in line with the core values of social work. There is widespread agreement that if intervention is to be effective then these must be underpinned by social perspectives that helps us to bring to our understanding of the social origins of mental disorder and the role that discrimination plays (SCIE, research briefing no 26, 2008). Social workers, after suitable post-qualifying training, can be a major part of such procedures and can also be involved in other aspects such as providing advocacy, reports for tribunals, arranging diversion into community resources, etc.

ACTIVITY 1.4

Think of a situation where, in practical terms, you will have to take culture into account when working with someone from a black or minority ethnic background.

COMMENT

There will be lots of examples that you could give and one is when compiling a Social Circumstances Report for a Mental Health Tribunal. Tribunals take place when someone has been detained in a psychiatric facility and wishes to appeal against this detention. The Tribunals consider various reports including ones compiled by social workers. These are formal reports that are presented to the Tribunal and they are a part of the mechanism by which compulsorily detained patients can be discharged from hospital. These reports provide the Tribunal with the cultural background of the service user and describe past patterns of behaviour that can help to determine the likely success of aftercare, together with other salient details such as accommodation and employment opportunities.

The Mental Health Act Code of Practice sets out as a guiding principle that all people should be respected for their:

> ... *diverse backgrounds as individuals and be assured that account will be taken of their age, gender, sexual orientation, social, ethnic, cultural and religious background, but that general assumptions will not be made on the basis of any one of these characteristics.*

(DoH, 1999, p.3)

This latter point is especially relevant as there is a risk of assuming cultural stereo-types, which can not only cause offence but can be widely misleading. In any event understanding someone's culture is only a first step towards anti-oppressive practice.

Are black and minority ethnic people the only community who get poorer services than the majority population? The answer is a qualified no! Other groups include older people, children and adolescents, women and people who are deaf. All these groups are covered in this book, but working with mental health users who are deaf raises some interesting parallels with working with black and minority ethnic users, as well as some challenges for you to face in your practice.

Deaf people and mental health

CASE STUDY

There are limited specialist services available for deaf people who have severe mental ill-ness. This was highlighted by the Independent Inquiry into the care and treatment of Daniel Joseph (Mischon, 2000), which was commissioned by some of the London Health Authorities. Daniel was profoundly deaf and was admitted to hospital from the courts having been made subject to a hospital order with restrictions after pleading guilty to man-slaughter with diminished responsibility. Concern over his treatment resulted in successive governments consulting about services across the spectrum for service users who are deaf.

People who are deaf, like black and minority ethnic people, report that mental health ser-vices are difficult to access and often do not cater for their specific needs. To raise our awareness of the specific needs of minority communities the Department of Health consul-tation paper *A Sign of the Times: Modernising mental health services for people who are deaf* (DoH, 2002) is worth consulting. Developing awareness of specific communities is an important, but only a first, step towards developing appropriate and responsive services.

The Royal National Institute for Deaf People estimates that there are eight million people who suffer from hearing loss, often associated with ageing, and that there are about 50,000 people for whom British Sign Language is their first and preferred language (RNID, 2003).

Members of the deaf community experience mental health problems just like people from any other community. However because of the difference in language and culture between those who are assessing deaf service users and the service users themselves, misdiagnosis can result and as a consequence deaf people can receive services and treatment that are inappropriate. Good practice needs to take into consideration the requirements of the Equality Act 2010 (DoH, 2010) which makes it clear that mental health services have to take reasonable steps to facilitate the uptake of services by people who are deaf and who have mental health problems (sometimes referred to as people with dual diagnosis). This includes the use of an interpreter at the various stages of assessment and provision of services.

Culture is a central feature of a person's identity and that at the very least must be taken into consideration when working with service users from black and minority ethnic communities or when working with service users who are deaf.

Does the relative social exclusion that deaf people experience contribute to their mental health problems? This is reported as being a factor in the relationship between the psychological health of deaf people and their subsequent call upon mental health services. In other words being deaf might increase your vulnerability to mental health problems (Ridgeway, 1997). In Chapter 2 explanations are given of the cause and manifestation of mental health problems and in particular the role that stress plays in mental health.

Until recently mental health services seemed to be based around the assumptions that users were all from a hearing population that is predominantly white British. Both of these assumptions are well off the mark and need to be challenged and changed. To meet the NSF Standard One services need to be provided that are sensitised to the needs of different people. In reality the respect for the person's cultural identity is the predominant value that ought to underpin your practice.

The Case Study below shows how services can respond in an ideal way. However, having a person who can effectively communicate in the same language as the service user is often a matter of luck and there is a need for more services of this nature. A deaf person who communicates through sign language is likely to find that being in an environment where fluent signers are is more conducive to their recovery than being in a hearing world. Of course once the specialist worker leaves the prison Shaz is left still having to cope with the traumas of prison, which is essentially a hearing world. This still leaves you having to explore with Shaz and the interpreter what specific needs she might have in respect to her deafness.

CASE STUDY

Shaz is a deaf person who lives alone and, at the age of 32, has very few connections with the deaf community. She is a fluent user of British Sign Language but since h   and to prison on theft charges her health has suffered. Over the last ten years or s treated for depression and has taken anti-depressants. The stress of bei caused her more distress to the extent that she would like to see a socia the prison service does not have a person who can sign and therefore side specialist support. By chance the local community mental health of staff who can sign and she accompanies the social worker to th an assessment with the prison doctor.

Learning disability and mental health

People who have a learning disability can experience a range of mental health problems just like the rest of us. However, the presence of learning disability may prevent professionals and carers recognising the symptoms of mental health problems such as depression. It is important for carers and professionals to look beyond stereotypes and seek explanations for behaviour that has typically changed. Finding out what is wrong will call for quality communication and observation skills and working in a partnership with carers and service users. There are some informative guides published by the Royal College of Psychiatrists and the likes of MENCAP, most of which you can download from their websites.

There are few research and evaluation studies in the field of learning disability and mental health – dual diagnosis is the technical term often used. This tends to maintain this important area as low priority yet Government policy expounded in the White Paper *Valuing People* urges people with learning difficulties to use mainstream NHS services (DoH, 2001). This of course includes mental health services.

The coexistence of mental health problems alongside learning disability may be one of the explanations of the existence of challenging behaviour. Such behaviour may not be a characteristic of learning disability but may be as a result of mental health problems. This is a theme that Moss picks up in his article in the *British Journal of Psychiatry*, which showed that there was 'some evidence for a statistical association between challenging behaviour and psychiatric disorder' (Moss, 2000, p.454). It concluded that depression was four times more prevalent in people with learning disability who exhibited challenging behaviour than for people with learning disability itself. This finding, although needing to be treated with some caution, is important as depression is so often overlooked in people with learning disability.

Working with service users who have this form of dual diagnosis often will mean mobilising community resources to provide support and connection with others in the community. This idea of connectedness is described by Peter Gilbert: 'Mental distress and mental illness is so often about a disconnection, false connections or an over concentration on one aspect of our lives' (2003, p.22). Like any other service user you as a social worker will want to access the whole person and how they draw support or otherwise from their families, carers and the community. Facilitating better connections within the community may be the most appropriate intervention that you can make.

Culturally competent practice: transforming social work

Cultural competence is a bringing together of some of the big ideas covered in this chapter. It is a combination of:

- awareness;
- nowledge of anti-oppressive practice;

- values-based practice;

- interpersonal skills that will provide you with the basic building blocks of a practice that is appropriate; and

- sensitivity to working with service users who may not always be from your own culture.

A culturally competent service can be defined as one that is perceived by minority ethnic users as being appropriate to their cultural and religious beliefs and responsive to their needs.

CASE STUDY

Christopher Clunis – inadequate care and treatment?

Christopher Clunis is a young African-Caribbean man who had a history of severe mental illness. He had been diagnosed as having paranoid schizophrenia when he lived in Jamaica. In December 1992 he attacked and killed Jonathan Zito who was completely unknown to him.

The subsequent Inquiry has been widely reported and some of the findings reveal the perils of professional practice that is not culturally relevant.

The Inquiry team concluded that:

> The added factor of his blackness may have contributed to the diffident manner in which some professionals treated him and it may have caused them to defer against his best interests, to his own expressed wishes.

(Ritchie et al., 1994, p.4)

and

> Young black males should not be type-cast as suffering from schizophrenia unless the clinical indications warrant it and clinicians and others who care for black mentally ill people should not be too ready to ascribe odd behaviour to the abuse of drugs.

(Ritchie et al., 1994, p.129)

This case study shows the extent to which stereotypical views can permeate professional practice and it highlights the dangers of seeing people only by the colour of their skin. Looking beyond this in a critical manner is the hallmark of good practice. At this point it is appropriate to examine the ways in which our practice can be transformed.

It should be clear that services need to become more relevant to the needs of black and minority ethnic groups and other minority groups such as people who are deaf. Service users frequently point out that the services that they are receiving show little understanding of their culture. But changing this is not a simple matter. You also need to recognise that this is a sensitive issue influenced by your own ethnicity and skin colour. Social workers who are skilled in anti-oppressive practice and using a values-based practice approach are clearly further on than those who are not, but there is no room for complacency as many of the explanations of service variability show that racism permeates organisations.

It is questionable whether we can be competent in cultures that are not our own and, in any case, the range of diverse cultures in the UK makes competence in all cultures an unrealistic proposition. An alternative to understanding different cultures is to recruit more social workers and other professionals from these minority communities to ensure cultural congruence or, in other words, proportionate representation of professionals from all groups. However, this can only be a limited strategy, for although positive action strategies when recruiting staff and adopting equal opportunities interview methods are vitally important, they are in themselves insufficient.

But what if you are a black social worker working with white service users or the other way around? What kind of approach can you adopt? To what extent do your stereotypes distort your assessment and decision-making processes? The National Institute for Mental Health England (NIMHE) has recommended that all staff working in this area receive compulsory training in cultural awareness to help eradicate racism and discrimination. Although there are many such courses around, quite a few of these promote awareness rather than competency. Awareness is just one stage in developing culturally competent practice.

Components of culturally competent practice

The idea of being able to work with a diverse range of cultures is not entirely new but has gained momentum and acceptance of late. Walker (2003) uses the idea of cultural competence building on the work of Kim (1995), while Patel et al. in *Engaging and Changing* (2003) refer to practice as being 'culturally sensitive', whereas Fulford (in MHAC 10th Biennial 2001–2003) describes 'value based practice'. Some of the common themes are blended together into five components of culturally competent practice and each of these is explored below.

Capacity for your own cultural awareness
This should start with an honest understanding of your own culture and the impact that this has on your professional practice. You need to be aware of your own attitudes, values and beliefs before you can be aware of the attitudes and beliefs of others.

Capacity for awareness of other cultures
It is a widely held view that self-awareness is one of the core components of a practice that is culturally competent (O'Hagan, 2001; Poole, 1998, etc.) but after that it is necessary for you to develop your own capacity for understanding the other cultures and putting this understanding into practice. This requires you to make a realistic assessment of your knowledge and understanding of working with people and of their cultures.

Understanding of diversity and difference

Community engagement is currently being promoted as the main way that professionals can increase their understanding of specific needs of communities. Social workers should respect diversity and build upon people's strengths and the collective strengths of the communities. Effective work with and across cultures requires that you understand and value difference both at the individual and at the community level. This also means recognising and accepting your own personal and professional limitations.

Transferring skills from one service user culture to another

At the heart of much of professional practice is the idea that skills that are learned from work with one type of problem can be transferred to another. This means that the skills that you have in assessing white people who have depression can also be used when working with Asian people who have depression. But as we have seen earlier, effective assessment requires you to understand the context in which the person is living. However, social work skills such as empowering practice are key components of this transforming practice.

Being able to recognise the impact of structural racism and discrimination

The Health and Social Care Act 2012 has at its centre the wellbeing of the individual and that local authorities must promote the individual's wellbeing in all decisions made with and about them. 'Wellbeing' is described in terms of the most important outcomes for people who use care and support for carers. This means that all providers of mental health services, including GPs and primary care workers, will be involved in some way or other in helping to deliver a service that is culturally appropriate and responsive to all groups in society.

Is it possible to achieve cultural competence?

The action plan called Delivering Race Equality in Mental Health Care, was the main driver behind the attempt to achieve a culturally more responsive and capable workforce. An interesting article in the *Guardian* should give cause for some healthy scepticism, a small extract of which follows:

> *Joanna Bennett, who leads research on workforce development at the Sainsbury Centre for Mental Health, has completed a review of race-related training and thinks that the picture is of 'a lot of fragmentation, different approaches and different models'. She says: 'There is no agreed definition of cultural competence and no evidence that it works in producing better services for black and minority ethnic users. We should be looking at structural processes and power relationships in the way services are delivered.'*

Bennett, a psychiatric nurse and former lecturer in mental health at Middlesex University, is the sister of David Bennett who died while in the care of mental health services. In evidence to the Inquiry into his death, she warned against services focusing on 'cultural matching' in favour of staff spending more time talking to patients and their families. Taking time to respect an individual, and ask what was troubling him and what he needed, was likely to be more effective than *talking about culture, ethnicity and cultural competence* (*Guardian*, Wednesday, 12 April 2006).

The significance of the above is that following the Inquiry into the death of Bennett, who had schizophrenia and who died during a restraint procedure at a medium secure unit, training for cultural competence was one of the high priority training recommendations. This followed the discovery during the Inquiry that very little attempt had been made to understand let alone relate to the racial and cultural needs of David Bennett.

Achieving cultural competence may well require more than individuals alone can achieve although, as Joanna Bennett points out, getting the basis right will go a long way towards providing a more user-focused service.

Promoting your own mental health

As you go through your course you are likely to be living a multitude of roles and having to meet numerous deadlines and expectations. These could include working to supplement your bursary or grant; balancing family life with college demands; worry about passing assignments and much more. Stress plays a big part in our own mental health and concern has risen in recent years over the increase in reported mental health problems for students in colleges and universities. In my experience social work students are no different from the majority of students studying on a variety of courses.

Students come to study at UK universities from all over the world and as a consequence the student community is as diverse as if not more so than the community at large. While many students can draw upon a range of personal resources, some are a long way from the support systems that have previously nurtured them. There are cultural differences, which also may mean that they are unwilling to talk about personal issues with comparative strangers. It could also be that those who could offer help and may be concerned do not recognise the signs or mistakenly interpret these signs as cultural differences.

It might be that you recognise some of these elements in yourself and that you are reluctant to seek help, partly because of the possible impact on your studies. If this is getting to be a serious problem you should seek help as social work is a stressful career and you need early on to develop strategies that will enhance your own mental health for dealing with such stresses.

It is unlawful for universities to treat students with mental health problems or physical difficulties, that have a substantial, adverse and long-term (more than 12 months) effect on the student's ability to carry out normal day-to-day activity, less favourably by excluding them temporarily or permanently if this is due to their actual mental health. Consequently a university should not exclude a student if their disruptive behaviour is primarily caused by mental health that falls into the realm of the Equality Act 2010.

Stress busting tip

The boxes technique

Think of a problem that you are currently dealing with (or have been recently) that has been causing you some concern, and how your mind goes over and over the problem. If that happens to you it can become stressful and unproductive. It can also prevent you from getting on with other things as your mind is focused on seemingly difficult problems. In time if this continues it can produce stress and perhaps sleepless nights. This is one technique for controlling and organising these problems that has been tried and tested by many students over the years.

1. Close your eyes and imagine that your mind is divided into a series of boxes and that each box has a lid.

2. Take each problem and place it into its own box.

3. Firmly place a lid on each box.

4. You now have your problems under control.

5. Only allow yourself to remove one lid at a time.

6. You can now focus all your attention on your released problem.

7. You may feel some of the lids on the other boxes starting to rise, if so be firm and replace them telling yourself that you will focus upon them at a later time. Persistent lid risers need a heavy weight to be placed upon them.

8. This technique really does work better with practice and students report that it is a good stress buster.

RESEARCH SUMMARY

The Mental Health Foundation commissioned research to overview current research and mental health initiatives related to student mental health. Among the findings was that clinical depression was reported in 12% of male students and 15% of females. This is an increase over the last time such estimates were made in 1987.

Student counsellors also reported an increase in the proportion of students with severe mental health problems or disorder. At the extreme end suicide among students has risen from 2.4 per 100,000 to 9.7. This is over the ten-year period 1983–1993/4.

(Fox, P. et al. in mentalhealth.org.uk/page.cfm?pagecode=PBUP0211)

CHAPTER SUMMARY

We have seen the impact that values and ethics have on mental health social work. These values are set down by the professional bodies and, in the case of social work, by the Health Care Professions Council.

Transforming social work in the twenty-first century requires workers to be able to recognise their own prejudices and biases and to move beyond these to develop a practice that is culturally competent, demonstrated by the worker's awareness of the service user's

(Continued)

(Continued)

culture, including religion and traits. It also means looking after your own mental health and recognising that we all are susceptible to various mental health problems.

Transforming practice means also engaging in more than the rhetoric of anti-oppressive practice and value-based practice. It means demonstrating that these major ideas have influenced everyday mental health work. This means seeing the person not just as the mental health problem that they exhibit and not being influenced by stereotypes. Listening to what users have to say about their experiences is an important part of this process.

FURTHER READING

Department of Health (1999) *The Mental Health Act Code of Practice.* London: DoH.

Gives specific practice guidelines when working with service users who are detained in psychiatric hospitals or units. It covers a range of activities including medication, other forms of treatment, control and restraint and what constitutes an emergency. This is essential reading for those who intend to practise in a mental health setting. NHS Trusts are advised to ensure that all staff undertake training in the meaning of the Code.

Department of Health (October 2003) *Delivering Race Equality: A framework for action consultation document.* London: DoH.

A consultation document that sets out the 9 building blocks of improved practice for mental health services.

WEBSITES

The Internet Encyclopedia of Philosophy has several pages concerned with the field of ethics and is a good place to visit for more information about 'normative principles in applied ethics'. **www.utm.edu/research/iep/e/ethics.htm**

Fox, P. et al. in **mentalhealth.org.uk**

RNID: fact sheet Introducing British Sign Language can be download free from **www.ucl.ac.uk/ library**

Department of Health (2010) *Equity and Excellence: Liberating the NHS,* available at: **http://tinyurl.com/EquityExcellenceliberatingnhs**

Department of Health (2010) *A Vision for Adult Social Care: Capable communities and active citizens,* available at: **www.dh.gov.uk/en/Aboutus/Features/dh_121664**

Department of Health (2010) *Healthy Lives, Healthy People: Transparency in outcomes – Proposals for a public health outcomes framework,* available at: **http://tinyurl.com/ Publichealthoutcomesconsult**

www.odi.gov.uk/equalityact provides easy access to the **Equality Act 2010** with many examples of mental impairment.

The Mental Health Foundation provide information on different ethnic minority groups and their mental health and can be accessed at **www.mentalhealth.org.uk/help-information/mental-health-a-z/B/BME-communities/**

Chapter 2
Social work practice and mental health

A C H I E V I N G   A   S O C I A L   W O R K   D E G R E E

This chapter will help you to develop the following capabilities from the **Professional Capabilities Framework:**

- **Professionalism**
  Identify and behave as a professional social worker committed to professional development.

- **Values and ethics**
  Apply social work ethical principles and values to guide professional practice.

- **Diversity**
  Recognise diversity and apply anti-discriminatory and anti-oppressive principles in practice.

- **Knowledge**
  Apply knowledge of social sciences, law and social work practice theory.

- **Critical reflection and analysis**
  Apply critical reflection and analysis to inform and provide a rationale for professional decision-making.

- **Intervention and skills**
  Use judgement and authority to intervene with individuals, families and communities to promote independence, provide support and prevent harm, neglect and abuse.

It will also introduce you to the following standards as set out in the 2008 social work subject benchmark statement:

4.3   Defining principles.
5.0   Subject knowledge, understanding and skills.
5.1.1   Social work services, service users and carers.
5.1.2   Service delivery context.
5.1.4   Social work theory.

Introduction

The greatest happiness of the greatest number is the foundation of morals and legislation.

Jeremy Bentham (1832)

This chapter introduces you to what is meant by mental illness and mental health and starts with the concept of 'lived experience' using a brilliant book to anchor our understanding of mental health from the service user perspective. Arguably the dominant model of mental illness is medical, which is also explored here. The importance of understanding not only what various diagnoses mean but also the implications of adopting the medical model is assessed. A contrasting perspective that incorporates social differences including gender, ethnicity, and age is also explored. Overlaid onto these differences are the social structural explanations that revolve around social exclusion and isolation, which will build on the foundations, laid in Chapter 1. The overall approach is eclectic and pragmatic but bear in mind that this is not a medical text and you should use this text to guide your study rather than as a sole resource.

What is meant by mental illness and mental health?

The first point that needs to be made is that there are different terms currently used to describe the same thing. For example you will hear terms such as mental distress, mental illness, mental disorder, mental health problems, mental health challenges, all used by students and professionals.

In this book the following terms are used.

Mental disorder is a broad term that covers any significant departure from a state of 'normal' health and includes diseases and illness. These include severe forms like schizophrenia and manic depression. Mental disorder implies that a state of 'normality' once existed and therefore offers the chance to work with the person to restore them to that state, and is usually a temporary condition.

Mental health is a difficult term to be categorical about as it is far more than the absence of illness. I suggest that it is about achieving your potential as a human being. People can have mental health problems, which are 'problems of everyday life' which just have to be got on with.

Learning disability (formerly known as mental handicap and before that as mental deficiency). With learning disability the individual's rate of progress is slower than for most and treatment is not about a cure, as this is a long-term, permanent condition, but about providing an environment in which the individual can achieve his or her potential.

RESEARCH SUMMARY

In 2007 the NHS Information Centre for Health and Social Care conducted the third survey, during the last 15 years, of the general population of psychiatric morbidity of adults years living in private households in Great Britain. In a wealth of fascinating data there is an interesting section about common mental disorders (CMDs), which are conditions that cause considerable emotional distress and interfere with daily life. CMDs include types of depression and anxiety states.

16.2% of adults met the diagnostic criteria for having a CMD in the week prior to the ONS interview and more than half of these people had a mixture of depression and anxiety states (9%). This is important as although less disabling than major psychotic disorders the greater prevalence of CMDs escalates the impact and therefore cost. You are very likely as a social worker to encounter people who are experiencing a CMD.

(Adult Psychiatric Morbidity in England, 2007: results of a household survey. NHS **https:// catalogue.ic.nhs.uk/publications/mental-health/surveys/adul-psyc-morb-res- hou-sur-eng-2007/adul-psyc-morb-res-hou-sur-eng-2007-rep.pdf.** This is a good place to look up data on a range of disorders.)

There are numerous perspectives about mental health and you need to acquire a good understanding of the various 'models' that are in current use. This means that you can evaluate one against the other and more importantly begin to put your prac- tice in an appropriate framework. To help your understanding the **social model** and the **medical model** are described as two key perspectives that inform work with ser- vice users who have mental disorder.

First we should consider from where the general public gets information about men- tal disorder: by and large, through the media. The lay perspective, as it might be called, is important and few studies have examined how people conceptualise mental health. One of the few studies in this area showed that mental illness and mental health are seen by the public as being part of the same continuum and have negative connotations.

ACTIVITY **2.1**

Messages in the media

Think about the media coverage of mental illness and jot down the memorable words. Can you remember the last time that you read an article that was using positive adjectives or celebrating the success of people with mental health problems? What terms are used to portray mental health? Does this portrayal vary from media source to media source, from tabloid to serious newspapers?

COMMENT

You may well have written down terms like 'nutter' or 'loony', which are in common use and have negative connotations. These are some of the ways that behaviours can become associated with certain labels and consequently become self-fulfilling prophecies. What are your views about this? Is calling someone a 'nutter' just a piece of harmless fun or does it bring with it unwanted labels?

Words that are used by the media and in particular the tabloid press are often associated with violence and risk. Even though the risk of a stranger who is mentally ill killing you is very small, some of the press coverage suggests that it is a common occurrence.

Finally you might find it interesting to look at coverage in the press over the next few weeks and compare different newspapers and, if you have the time, think about how you would rewrite the headline or sub-heads. Positive coverage and useful information can be found at the BBC website for example: **www.bbc.co.uk/ newsbeat/24804164**

Understanding mental health
The importance of lived experience

The lived experience of people with mental illness is of huge value as we, the professionals, try to understand mental health and to develop our own approach to working with people. Being able to walk in someone's shoes is so important. But people with mental health problems are, just like you and me, all very different and as a result we can meet people who manage chronic conditions so well that we hardly even know about this and of course there are those who are forced to live on the margins of society. One way is to look at the literature especially those where the author describes their journey. There are I am pleased to say far more than ever of such accounts. Maybe you already are familiar with these but if not a few minutes' search on organisations' websites such as the 'Black Dog Institute', 'Mind UK', 'beyondblue' will produce countless texts.

You may have seen the film *A Beautiful Mind* which recounts the moving story of the Nobel Prize winner John Nash who, as a leading academic at the Ivy League University of Princeton, suffered from schizophrenia and eventually with the support of family, colleagues and professionals learnt to mange his disease and make a pretty full recovery. This is a very visual story but you can also begin to understand what the experience of mental illness is by turning to the literature.

One of the books that I suggest you read is by Elyn Saks who is an eminent professor at the University of Southern California. The title is *The Center Cannot Hold,* published in 2007, and it follows on from texts like *Girl Interrupted* by Susanna Kaysen and *An Unquiet Mind* written by Kay Jamison. All recount in beautiful ways the journey that young women have made in and out of psychosis. But back to Elyn Saks' account of her mental health problems – a book that won one million dollars and universal accolades. It is also a book that offers fellow sufferers hope and helps professionals to understand the nature of her mental illness and what role they can play in helping the service user to manage and possibly recover. Professor Saks in 2009 was a recipient of a MacArthur Foundation fellowship and in autumn 2010 it was announced that the funds from the 'genius grant' were to be used to create the Saks Institute for Mental Health Law, Policy, and Ethics. The Institute spotlights one important mental health issue per academic year.

Saks' first episode came when she was a teen, growing up in the USA, with as she describes loving and caring parents. This is in line with the accepted wisdom that schizophrenia frequently starts in early adulthood (National Collaborating Centre for Mental Health, 2013; NHS Choices, 2010). It was the start of a very scary journey. She brilliantly describes her experience as if she was a 'sand castle with all of the sand sliding away in the receding surf. So that in the end there was no center(sic) to take things in and process them and view the world'. If Elyn's reality could change so suddenly for her it gives us a degree of insight into how realities are constructed in the first instance. She recounts during one period when walking back from school how she believed that houses in the neighbourhood were communicating thoughts to her. This decomposing of her reality is a common experience of people who have episodes of psychosis.

Later and when at Oxford University as a Marshall Scholar away from family and friends she became depressed, lonely and totally lost her appetite. She withdrew into herself believing that she wasn't to speak lest she spread 'evil' around the world. She began to think that people were talking about her and that she was receiving instructions about what to do. Mental automatism is a process used in psychiatry to understand how a person may feel that every action or thought is commented upon by a voice outside of them (Leader, 2012, p.43). In effect, for Elyn, she moved during her episode from observing reality to having reality talk back to her. Language that used to create one reality has now started to re-create a new and frightening reality. In this way language has started to function autonomously.

What is special about this writing is that it charts a journey that few of us will experience yet retains a positive approach about how despite still suffering from the symptoms of schizophrenia she has managed through therapy and medication to handle it well and still to continue her job and relationships.

The journey through mental illness is different for different people. Yet we all want the same things and have far more in common with each other than we have separated by the effects of mental illness. In making a diagnosis psychiatrists use guides like the DSM-5 as their 'bible' of diagnostic criteria but one consequence can be that the person ceases to be a unique individual and becomes a component of the treatment and services. This can be profoundly disabling and disempowering especially if you think your world is being controlled by others and not just external voices. Elyn describes her experience of being compulsorily detained, as 'It was horrifying it's demeaning and debilitating to have choice taken away in general, to be not respected as an autonomous agent' (interview with *TIME* accessed 19/10/2013: **http://conten. time.com/time/art/article/0,8599,1656592,00.html**)

The DSM-5 makes a distinction between mood disorders and thought disorders and consequently schizophrenia is a good example of a thought disorder characterised by psychosis. Psychosis is broadly understood as being out of touch with reality. The common understanding of schizophrenia is a 'split personality' which Elyn writes is a misunderstanding as in her case her mind was not split but shattered.

She explains that she is not wildly psychotic all the time and describes her positive symptoms, things that you have but do not want, for example delusions and hallucinations.

Negative symptoms would include some form of deficit like apathy or withdrawal. Not everyone will experience all of these symptoms.

So how did she manage her symptoms and turn out to be the brilliant professor that she is? Well the answer in part lies with the central role that medication has played and also the importance to her of talking therapy. Now often people with schizophrenia do not benefit from talking therapy but that is certainly not the case with her. For Elyn the opportunity on a regular basis to sit with someone and to feel safe when sharing very deep subjects proved invaluable. As she says, this gets to the heart of relationships and about who we are and how we relate to others – the very stuff of social work.

In a rich and readable book Elyn puts two important ideas alongside one another that she could be mentally ill and yet lead a rich and satisfying life. She is inspirational.

Listening to service users' experience of mental health, whether celebrity or just regular people, can help you to transform your understanding of what mental illness is and how best you can work to develop best practice. But these understandings need to be based on a critical and intellectual appreciation of social work. One that can be underpinned by shared values and incorporated into your professional life and work.

In my opinion it is important to ground your professional practice in an understanding of the lived experiences of people who experience mental illness and to be able to place this alongside our own lived experiences. This may sound strikingly obvious but by taking this approach it helps you to frame your practice as much more than a focus upon the narrowness of diagnosis and symptoms. Remember that people are much more than just a label like mentally ill. People are not schizophrenics but people first who have schizophrenia.

Explaining mental health

It is easy to see that there are two perspectives about what causes mental health:

- that held by the medical practitioners, which is essentially a biomedical or disease model;
- and that held by professionals like social workers, which looks at social causation and/or labelling as explanations.

This separation into one or the other model is probably only useful in an academic or research sense as the medical perspective dominates and other perspectives need to at least take this perspective on board. I have a great sympathy with the view that the mental health field, in fact perhaps social work itself, is riven with 'unhelpful binaries' (Bland, 2009); the use of binary is another more accurate way of saying opposites. Think about binaries in respect of mental health and how we use these notions to determine if someone is sane or insane, yet this is most likely a continuum along which we can all be located and a position that may change dependent upon time and circumstance. This use of binaries as explanatory concepts can help to understand how we sometimes get into tension between using a clinical or medicalised model as opposed to a social or critical model of understanding about mental health. What we use in universities, as a means of critical understanding, may well not transfer v the social work setting.

Although we now explore both these models you should consider them as theoretical ideas and remember that in order to be effective, social workers often have to work in the swampy low grounds of everyday practice. This is now explored.

The medical or clinical model

This is a medical perspective that is adopted by doctors and psychiatrists and is sometimes called the 'disease model'. The acceptance of this model gives credence to the claim that organic or biomedical causes will eventually be found for all forms of mental disorder. Although the psychiatric model dominates discourse about mental disorder, this is as much by accident as it is by virtue of its conceptual strength. Andrew Scull, in his book *Museums of Madness* (1979), describes how a transformation occurred from people being seen as eccentrics, village fools or possessed by the demon when, around 150 years ago, the state took control and the medical profession was employed to treat and manage mental disorder.

In contemporary practice social workers work alongside other health professionals including psychiatrists to deliver mental health services. At some point you will be involved in an assessment of what the service users' needs are, which may necessitate a diagnosis. However, the main focus for you will be in the areas of recovery, working with individuals and family to promote wellbeing and control over their lives. As a social worker you are used to working on the interface between service user and others where your work may be to promote equity and fairness as well as helping to challenge oppression and discrimination.

Assessment

As a social worker you are most likely to be involved in this early stage of assessment and treatment of mental disorder. Campbell (1999) suggests that social workers can only become competent when, as practitioners, they are able to synthesise interpersonal skills with theories and ideas about the causes of mental disorder. This is the case for all settings and aspects of the work. You may also be involved later in your career as an Approved Mental Health Professional (AMHP) or similar with specific responsibilities under the legislation to assess a service user for whom compulsory admission to hospital may be the last resort. This is covered in the chapter on legal issues. An in-depth assessment would need to include some or all of the following:

- previous history of mental health problems or difficulties;
- service user self-assessment of their difficulties;
- cultural and religious aspects;
- employment status;

- relationship strengths and weaknesses;

- substance use or misuse including drug and alcohol use.

The importance of this approach is to identify what would be considered to be the most effective way of proceeding with the service user. The aim is to work in a manner that the service user would describe as culturally sensitive and which focuses upon the service user's strengths rather than deficits. Service users who have experienced mental health problems may have also experienced what works for them and your task may be one of mobilising resources to help them deal with their problems.

For those service users who are clearly presenting with behaviours that are likely to need more specialist services and possible medication, a referral to the GP and then to psychiatric services would be appropriate and even necessary.

Diagnosis

A diagnosis of mental disorder is always given by a doctor who is usually also a psychiatrist. It should emerge out of considerable contact between the doctor and the service user. Assessment as described above is a process of collecting information that will assist in the making of a diagnosis. Conventionally the language of psychiatry replaces 'mental disorder' with the term 'mental illness' and 'service user' with 'patient'. Psychiatrists are trained to use a phenomenological approach, or in other words they try to establish a pattern of signs and symptoms. This helps to distinguish between people who are eccentric, unusual or who have only occasional symptoms from those whose symptoms indicate more severe disorder.

To avoid variation in assessment between doctors it is common to use one of a number of psychiatric assessment tools or interview schedules. These have all been standardised, a process by which the reliability of these tools is established. They help the psychiatrist to assess the presence of certain symptoms which act as signposts to effective diagnosis. The schedules include the **Present State Examination** (**PSE**), which has 40 components to it, or the more commonly used **Beck Depression Inventory.**

The importance of a diagnosis is that it:

- acts as a pathway to more specialised care and treatment;

- is a process in which most patients have faith (sometimes in spite of the evidence);

- can mobilise support from other agencies such as housing and income benefit for those in need;

- should involve other professional views being sought, including those of social workers;

- should occur over a period of time and not be an assessment that is made over a few days, but rather weeks or even months.

However, service users seldom report the diagnostic process as being empowering and often complain that their views are seldom sought except as signposts to a diagnosis.

Classification of mental disorders

Classification is an important step in the diagnosis of mental disorder. Mental disorder is broken down into various classifications that represent groups or syndromes of symptoms or phenomena. Thus if a series of symptoms fits into a recognised pattern they can be classified as, for example, schizophrenia and a diagnosis made. A diagnosis is a shorthand version of what the psychiatrist believes to be wrong with the patient. Such classifications also enable treatment and outcomes to be better predicted. In the UK psychiatrists use one of two texts, either the **DSM-5** (American Psychiatric Association's Diagnostic and Statistical Manual of Mental disorders, 2013) or the **ICD-10** (International Classification of Diseases Volume 10 (World Health Organisation, 1992)). This has created two systems of psychiatric diagnosis and the possibility of unnecessary confusion and attempts will be made to achieve increased consistency between the forthcoming ICD-11 and DSM-5. Although as a social worker you will not be using these manuals to diagnose it is worth familiarising yourself with some of their main features. This will help you to understand the basis of a diagnosis.

The nature of this process is rigorous and great efforts have been made to try to ensure their validity and reliability. For example the ICD, published in 1992, but soon to be replaced, took nine years to prepare and was tested and included extensive field trials of the draft text in many countries (Eldergill, 1997). Even so they have been the subject of dispute over the years (Menninger, 1963) and remember that a diagnosis is only as good as the information on which it is based. You might want to think about how much these diagnoses are affected by social factors, societal values and historical context.

Although as a social worker you are usually not directly involved with the determination of a diagnosis, you will need to share the ownership of it when working as part of a multidisciplinary team. It is important that you have some understanding, at least of the main characteristics of the above and what the various treatment options are for each. You are also, more than most professionals, going to be involved in the complex interaction of the service user and their cultural and social background. For example with disorders like depression, which has a biological component to it, a combination of medication and social intervention is often the most effective treatment. However don't forget that assessment is not the same as diagnosis.

The limitations of the DSM-5 approach

There should be a health warning issued alongside the very expensive DSM-5, along the lines that strict adherence to this manual may be bad for your service user's health. This diagnostic manual is one of two in current use and as it has just been updated represents the march of the scientific approach towards the treatment of mental illness. It would be wrong to dismiss the medical profession's approach towards mental health for many advances have been made with pharmacology that have made a significant difference to the management of mental illness such as depression and schizophrenia.

Think back to Elyn Saks where she is clear that the continuing use by her of powerful anti-psychotic drugs is fundamental to her quality of life. But in her case this was also alongside regular psychodynamic support and counselling.

This focus on people rather than technology is a theme promulgated by psychiatrist Professor Tom Burns in his recent book *Our Necessary Shadow: The Nature and Meaning of Psychiatry* (2013) where he suggests that psychiatry is dependent upon the relationship that the psychiatrist and other professionals have with the service user. As he points out, the emotional labour that is required to work with service users that are demoralised and depressed or severely deluded is considerable and this in turn leads to a degree of over-optimism on the part of professionals, who anticipate complete recovery for many when this is but an outside chance.

Are we in danger of medicalising everyday life and are we searching for medical explanations that allow us to step back from the trials and tribulations that life possess? This is where the major criticism of the DSM-5 and its predecessors can be levelled, as the likes of Burns argue that it serves the needs of health insurance providers and drug manufacturers far more than it does the needs of people who have mental illness. It is no surprise that its origins is primarily in the USA where private medicine dominates the health sector. A search through the DSM-5 can be quite revealing and don't be surprised to find conditions that include caffeine intoxication and female sexual arousal disorder (FSAD). If there was ever a man for all seasons then this surely is a diagnostic manual for all seasons.

Treatment

There are different ways of treating users who have mental disorder. The effectiveness of such treatment depends upon the nature of the disorder and the skills of the people who are providing the treatment. These treatments are briefly discussed below. Every treatment option must have the risks weighed up alongside the possible benefits, for no treatment is without some cost and risk. Medical practitioners are trained first and foremost to do no harm to their patients. The dominant mode of treatment is medication but treatment also includes the following:

Psychosurgery
This is little used and then only for those with chronic conditions of obsessional and depressive disorders. It can only be given with the patient's informed consent, and Section 57 of the Mental Health Act (1983) applies to both informal and formal patients and provides additional safeguards. This is irreversible removal or destroying of brain tissue.

Electroconvulsive therapy (ECT)
ECT consists of administering an electric shock to patients who are sedated and is usually used when there has been an inadequate response to medication. It can be an effective treatment for depression, especially when this is accompanied by psychotic delusions. Patients are usually given a course of treatment of six to twelve applications.

Psychological

Psychological inputs are many and varied and include:

- behavioural therapy, which is based on learning theory;

- cognitive therapy, which focuses on incorrectly, learned behaviours;

- counselling which also has numerous variants;

- psychotherapy which also includes many variants;

- family therapy.

Alternative medicine

As yet many of the 'alternative therapies', although popular with service users, are not 'proven' by research. They include hypnotherapy, dance, acupuncture and herbal remedies, and can have a role to play in combination with other modes of treatment. As interest continues, some clinical trials have suggested that for moderate depression St John's Wort may be effective, and evidence suggests that exercise and lifestyle may also perform valuable protective functions.

Medication

Medication has become an important part of the treatment of mental disorder for many service users but it is not the only way of managing mental disorder. Medication works by either stopping the release of chemicals in the brain or by increasing the activity of certain parts of the brain. In the 1950s there was a 'pharmacological revolution' with the arrival of new forms of medical treatment including Chlorpromazine (Jones, 1993). This changed the lives of many patients with enduring mental illness in long-stay hospitals by giving them the opportunity to be treated in the community.

Today there is a 'new revolution' of 'atypical' anti-psychotic drugs, which have far fewer side effects than the previous ones and are also in many instances more effective. Some of the older medications caused amenorrhoea in women, which may have prevented long-term users from having children, whereas the main side effect of the new medication is significant weight gain. Medication is divided into six types, as shown in Table 2.1.

Table 2.1

Type	Example	Typical use
Anti-psychotics	Chlorpromazine, Risperidone and in treatment-resistant conditions Clozapine	Schizophrenia
Anti-depressants	Prozac (fluoxetine)	Depression
Anti-manic	Lithium	Mania
Anti-epileptic	Carbamazepine	Epilepsy
Anxiolytics	Diazepam	Anxiety states
Hypnotics	Temazepam	Insomnia

RESEARCH SUMMARY

Explaining the rise in antidepressant prescribing: a descriptive study using the general practice research database

An article in the British Medical Journal (BMJ) *explored the rise in the number between 1993 and 2005 of prescription items for anti-depression. Like other parts of the more developed world this has increased but not it seems because more people are becoming depressed but rather because more patients are on medication longer than before and this group consumes the most drugs.*

(Moore, M et al. (2009) Explaining the rise in antidepressant prescribing: a descriptive study using the general practice research database, BMJ 2009; 339 :b3999)

Understanding the major forms of mental disorder

The dilemma facing anyone who works with disturbed people is to be able to differentiate between 'normal' and 'abnormal' behaviour. The unusual behaviour or eccentricities of people are what make life so interesting and we should value such diversity. Clearly though there is a point beyond which the eccentric becomes markedly disordered and the person is in need of help. The main disorders that you will come across are described in the next part of this chapter.

Schizophrenia

Schizophrenia is a complex thought disorder with a number of variants, although the prognosis is well understood by specialists. It is a neuropsychiatric disorder where a number of factors may have impacted upon the central nervous system and which results in a cluster of symptoms that are classified as schizophrenia. There is a view that schizophrenia is a collection of different illness rather than a single entity, which helps to understand why there are seemingly so many different manifestations of schizophrenia. It is commonly thought, incorrectly, by the general public to be associated with dangerousness and extreme madness and thus carries a stigma, which other diagnoses do not (Eldergill, 1997).

Symptoms may be acute but the condition is usually chronic. There are frequent periods of low level affect followed by acute episodes resulting in drops in social and cognitive functioning. Symptoms can include the following.

Hallucinations
These are problems to do with sensory perception, which are real for the person who experiences them. They include: auditory hallucinations (including hearing voices) and somatic hallucinations (the user believes that they are experiencing phenomena like electricity running through their body).

Delusions

These are beliefs which are considered bizarre, are clearly not supported by the available evidence yet are held in an unshakable manner by the person. Delusions can be part of systematic thought or appear to be completely random. These are usually culturally specific, hence in the UK some people are deluded into grandiose thinking, believing that they are related to the royal family or are relatives of the prime minister.

Interference with thought

Thought insertion is a form of delusion involving the belief that someone else's thoughts can be placed in the person's mind. This can also be perceived as a form of thought control where it is believed that someone outside is controlling your thoughts, or thought broadcast where you believe that your private thoughts are being broadcast to the general public.

Schizophrenia affects about 1% of the population. The onset is usually during adolescence or early adulthood but can occur later on in life. Before an accurate diagnosis is made the symptoms should have been noted over at least six months and must include at least one active psychotic phase. Early recognition and treatment significantly improves the overall prognosis for the user, consequently social workers should be aware of this and raise this diagnosis as a possibility rather than waiting. Early medication can alter the course of schizophrenia (Frangou and Bryne, 2000).

Features associated with schizophrenia

Episodes may consist of three phases in which 'normal functioning' is interrupted as follows:

1. **Pre-onset or prodromal phase** in which noticeable changes occur including social isolation, difficulty in functioning, odd behaviour, blunted affect, bizarre ideas, and lack of energy. Friends and relatives may describe the person's behaviour during this phase, as 'he/she is not the same person as he/she was'.

2. **Onset or active phase** is where the behaviours and thoughts are acutely psychotic and often include delusions, which are false or irrational beliefs; hallucinations in which the most common is hearing voices; incoherence; belief that others can read your mind or hear your innermost thoughts and feelings of persecution. These need to be present for at least a week and can be the result of some stressful psycho-social event.

3. **Residual phase** is very similar to the pre-onset phase except that the person may experience negative affect and a flattening of emotions. They could still be hearing voices or other psychotic features but these are less strong.

Treatment and management

The usual treatment regime is a combination of medication and psycho-social interventions. While medication does not 'cure' it can dramatically correct serious and abnormal phenomena such as hallucinations or delusions.

The over-representation of young African-Caribbean males who are diagnosed as having schizophrenia is of major concern and points to the lack of culturally sensitive practice (see Chapter 1).

43

What is the social work role?

Social work intervention can include:

- education with the service user and their family;

- helping to arrange appropriate low stress accommodation;

- networking with the service user to provide community support;

- the use of behavioural techniques to modify behaviours;

- encouraging compliance with medication;

- acting as an advocate for the service user where appropriate.

What is the outlook or prognosis for people with schizophrenia?

About one-third of people who are diagnosed with schizophrenia will completely recover but for the remainder the outlook is one that will include at least one more episode, and for some schizophrenia will turn into a major challenge for them and their families or carers. The picture is much better than it was 20 years ago, in large part due to more effective interventions and the emergence of the newer anti-psychotic drugs that have fewer side effects than their predecessors.

(Chapter 7 has an illustrative example about schizophrenia.)

Mood disorders: depression

Depression is a group of mental disorders that can affect many of us at some point in our lives. It can affect anyone, at any age, and is often overlooked among the very young and the elderly. Depression is a mood disorder characterised by mood change that explains why this disorder is termed a mood or affective disorder. There are different types of depression including manic depression, post-natal depression and clinical or major depression that affect about 3–4% of the population in any one year. More females are affected than males.

Depression is categorised into three levels of severity: mild, moderate or severe. The ICD-10 is a good source for further information about these levels. However, in essence the mild level allows users to receive treatment from their GPs and to continue with much of their lives; the moderate sees the user continuing their social, work or domestic lives with increased difficulty and with the severe it is unlikely that the user will be able to live a 'normal' life and suicide is a distinct risk.

Features associated with depression

Anyone can suffer from depression from time to time and it only becomes of clinical interest when the severity increases or the duration of the episode is longer than might be expected. Assessment is carried out using some psychiatric rating scales (Beck's Depression Inventory).

Treatment and management

A range of treatments is possible depending upon the severity of the disorder. Among the treatments indicated are courses of anti-depressant medications, including the use of Prozac, which interacts with the neuro-chemical pathways both in the brain and elsewhere in the body. The use of medication is often combined with psycho-social intervention to provide effective treatment. In severe depression it is important to take the risk of suicide seriously and to consult about risk with your medical colleagues. The user should always be asked about suicide, and where they exhibit plans for suicide or preoccupation with it then this should be seen as clear intent and action taken. (See Chapter 6 for an example on suicide.)

What is the social work role?

Social work interventions can include:

- identification of risk;

- management of risk;

- encouraging service users to take prescribed medication;

- individual counselling;

- cognitive behavioural therapy (CBT);

- referring for specialist psychotherapy;

- community networking.

Mood disorder: bipolar affective disorder (manic depression)

This is a mood disorder in which the person can feel intermittently depressed and occasionally elated. In the ICD mania and depression are cited as opposite ends of the same spectrum, hence the term bipolar. Mania is characterised by extreme elevation of mood and physical and mental energy and activity. It can exist in its own right (uni-polar) but usually it is accompanied by at least one episode of depression. Because during mania the user believes that he/she is well, treatment is difficult and the social and financial consequences can be damaging as the person squanders their money or does other similar extravagances. Consequently hospital in-patient treatment may be required in order for the user's mood to return to normal.

The main medication is lithium although there are other medications available. This is a mood stabiliser that works by controlling the extent of racing thoughts rather than sedation, and although it takes a few days to work it does seem to prevent a swing into depression. It is particularly effective in the prevention of relapse among patients who have previously been diagnosed.

Dual diagnosis

The term dual diagnosis covers a spectrum of disorders that combine with mental disorder. While these can include mental disorder and learning disability they generally refer to mental disorder and substance abuse. This latter category has presented acute wards in hospitals with some of the most serious of challenges. In urban areas many of the patients admitted to hospital have experience of substance misuse, a habit which some try to continue while they are on the ward. The most common forms of misuse are drugs and alcohol.

The relationship between these conditions and the interactive effect are complex. These include:

- mental disorder that precipitated substance abuse;
- mental disorder, which is worsened by the overlay of substance abuse;
- intoxication and/or substance abuse, which results in psychological symptoms;
- withdrawal of substance abuse that results in psychiatric symptoms.

(Adapted from *Dual Diagnosis Good Practice Guide*, DoH, 2002)

Jacqui Smith, the then Minister for Health, said in April 2002

> *All too often people with 'dual diagnosis' – the twin problems of severe mental illness combined with drug and alcohol problems – have fallen between two stools, and been unable to find the help that they need from either mental health or substance misuse services.*

(Launch of the Acute In-Patient Care and Dual Diagnosis guidance, Jacqui Smith, 2002)

The National Office of Statistics demonstrated high levels of drug use in prisons, suggesting that 10% of remand prisoners had a moderate drug dependency, 40% had a severe dependency and among remand prisoners who were substance abusers over 75% had mental health problems (in *Dual Diagnosis Good Practice Guide*, 2002).

There is an increased risk of suicide for people with dual diagnosis and as substance misuse is becoming more common it should always be looked for in assessments.

Treatment can involve motivational interviewing, assertive outreach, individual counselling and most importantly providing an integrated service. Associated with drug and alcohol abuse are increased physical health problems.

What is the social work role?
Social work interventions can include:

- identification of risk;
- management of risk;
- encouraging service users to take prescribed medication;
- cognitive behavioural therapy (CBT);
- community networking;
- liaison with other agencies and professionals.

Organic disorders

The organic disorders considered here are those associated with increasing age, most notably dementia. However don't forget that older people can also experience depression and other mental disorders in much the same way as their younger counterparts. The presence of depression in older people should be actively looked for and the person's presentation can mean that organic disorder is masked behind other mental disorders. For example approximately one person in five suffers from depression when they are over 60 and about one in ten actually develops depression after they have reached retirement age. There is a heightened risk of suicide among older people with depression.

Alzheimer's disease is a degenerative disease where the brain has been irreversibly damaged. Similar symptoms can also occur through excessive and prolonged consumption of alcohol or as a result of traumatic injury, a stroke or misuse of drugs. Sometimes the impairment can be acute and recovery is possible. In the case of Alzheimer's disease, which is considered to be a chronic condition, the brain progressively degenerates which results in impaired intellect, disorientation and eventually death.

Features associated with Alzheimer's

It is important to distinguish between the 'normal' effects of ageing and the development of a progressive disorder like Alzheimer's. We all suffer the loss of brain cells as we age but with this disorder cell loss is more rapid and profound than would be expected. The rate of degeneration does vary but it is usual for this to get more rapid as the disorder progresses.

Treatment and management

The early stages can be accompanied by depression, anxiety and severe sleep disturbance as the service user may have insight into the progressive nature of this disorder. Older people do better in familiar surroundings than in institutional care, but admission to residential care may be necessary where there is significant risk of self-neglect. The NHS will introduce a new brain scanning technique gradually from 2013 that will allow doctors to rule out a patient having Alzheimer's — the most common form of the disease — or the chance that it will develop within five years. This is important as it represents the first test that can be carried out while the person is alive. The scan was developed by scientists in London and is administered by giving a patient, exhibiting signs of dementia, a small amount of a radioactive substance, which will allow amyloid plaques to show up in a brain scan.

The presence of these plaques in the brain is one of the main signs of Alzheimer's, although it does not make the disease inevitable, so doctors using the test would be sure of giving a patient the all clear only if the plaques were absent. This marks a big improvement on the present assessment of function which results in about one in five patients being wrongly diagnosed with all of the attendant worries and anxieties that this can cause for all concerned.

What is the social work role?

Social workers will work as part of a team that ideally will provide a system of care that encompasses the provision of support services of different kinds to the user and their carers, depending on their level of need. The social work role includes arranging welfare benefits, providing information and explanation of the user's situation to family, neighbours and others, arranging and financing social support systems and eventually specialist nursing care if necessary (Eldergill, 1997).

Defining dementia

The national dementia strategy document is a good place to start to look for an understandable definition of dementia:

> The term 'dementia' is used to describe a syndrome which may be caused by a number of illnesses in which there is progressive decline in multiple areas of function, including decline in memory, reasoning, communication skills and the ability to carry out daily activities. Alongside this decline, individuals may develop behavioural and psychological symptoms such as depression, psychosis, aggression and wandering, which cause problems in themselves, which complicate care, and which can occur at any stage of the illness.

> The causes of these illnesses are not well understood to date but they all result in structural and chemical changes in the brain leading to the death of brain tissue. The main sub-types of dementia are: Alzheimer's disease, vascular dementia, mixtures of these two pathologies ('mixed dementia') and rarer types such as Lewy body dementia, dementia in Parkinson's disease and fronto-temporal dementia. The term 'Alzheimer's disease' is used sometimes as a shorthand term to cover all forms of dementia.

> The dementias all share the same devastating impact on those affected and their family carers. Dementias affect all in society irrespective of gender, ethnicity and class. They can affect adults of working age as well as older adults. People with learning disabilities are a group at particular risk. This Strategy is designed to address the needs of all people with dementia, no matter of what type, age, ethnic origin or social status.

> (DOH, 2009, p.16)

The impact of dementia

Dementia is one of the most severe and devastating disorders we face. It is also very common. Dementia is predominantly a disorder of later life, but there are at least 15,000 people under the age of 65 who have the illness. The illness itself can have a devastating impact on the lives of all concerned. This can be especially hard on primary carers often old and frail themselves. Even though the prognosis for people with dementia is generally about 7–12 years this can have a major impact on the families and loved ones.

But all is not gloom and despair and a great deal can be done and of course should be done to help people with dementia. The early diagnosis is one step that is being encouraged and this in turn will help people with dementia and their family carers to receive treatment, care and support and knowledge of the illness that will enable them to live the best quality of life that is possible. One of the advantages of early diagnosis is that it empowers people to make informed choices. If on the other hand a diagnosis is made well into dementia, or not even at all, informed plans for their future become irrelevant and they are denied the potential that help, support and treatments (social and psychological, as well as pharmacological) can offer.

What is the role of social workers with people who have dementia?

Although much of the literature focuses upon the organic nature of dementia, among the major effects are those on social and relationships. The challenge facing all services is high and the challenge is to provide fully resourced social work services that are capable of meeting the complex needs of older people and reducing age-related discrimination. Professor Tom Kitwood developed as long ago as the 1960s a 'person–centred care' approach. This is a positive way of working that means even if a person with dementia may lose their personhood this can be maintained through relationships with other people. One of his key points was that people are different and it is helpful to understand their personal history which in turn enables social workers and carers to understand what triggers changes in patient behaviour. He gives an example of someone shouting and getting very agitated when people don't sit down, realising that this person used to be a teacher enables care workers to tailor their contacts that reduce stress and agitation. There are also positive ways in which connection can be made with the person with dementia that would include sensory stimulation such as music and smells and doing something which the person really enjoys.

Figure 2.1 shows the relationship between the key aspects of a person's life and their wellbeing and illustrates the energies and skills a care worker needs to use when working with a person with dementia. Thus the social work role may involve in working with the person and with the family and significant others. In the early stages it may be about adjusting to the situation and involve you working with nurses and the GP to help the person and their family understand the nature of dementia and the journey that they are emabarking upon.

Figure 2.1   Person-centred care and adaptation of Kitwood's Dementia Reconsidered (1997)

According to the best estimates available, care home placement of people with dementia costs the UK £7 billion per year with two-thirds paid by social services and one-third by older people and their families themselves. While it is clearly the case that some people will need and benefit from admission to care homes, and that this can be a positive choice, there is also a strong quality argument for the prevention of unnecessary institutionalisation. People with dementia generally want to stay in their own homes, as do their carers.

(*Living Well With Dementia: a national dementia strategy*, 2009, p.34)

Research has pointed out that individuals and carers want to have people to whom they can talk and explore their feelings as well as getting practice advice and guidance.

...'someone to be with us on the journey'. Current health and social care services normally discharge individuals once the case is stable and the care package is being delivered. This is almost always perceived negatively by people with dementia and their carers, who, faced with a serious illness where there is inevitable long-term decline and increase in dependency, want to feel that there is continuing support available to them when they need it.

(*Living Well With Dementia: a national dementia strategy*, 2009, p.40)

There is also the practice wisdom that people in the early stages of dementia do well with physical rehabilitation and being involved in regular physical and mental stimulation.

Dementia: a worldwide response?

In December 2013 the G8 held a dementia summit to see if there could be a global response to what has been variously described as a 'looming epidemic', a 'tsunami' and a 'ticking time bomb' (*Guardian*, 11 December 2013). The reason for such statements is the suggestion that 34 million of us worldwide have the disease now with this to triple by 2050 (**www.who.int/features/factfiles/dementia/en/**). In the UK there are 800,000 people with dementia that in 2013 cost an estimated £23bn. The reality is that dementia will, if not already, touch every family in the UK. There is no cure at present for dementia and treatments at best postpone the inevitable, which in turn has prompted the G8 to begin to draw up a 'global action plan' in the hope and perhaps expectation that if a massive focused effort could be developed ways could be found to prevent dementia becoming an inevitable part of the ageing process. In the short to medium term the aim is to double research in the UK and to mirror the massive efforts made in the drive to find cures for cancer. It is well worth keeping an eye on the progress of this initiative and let's hope that fine words don't stay just that and action occurs.

Critical psychiatry

While for the last 50 years the medical model has dominated the explanatory landscape there have been pockets of disaffection that have gained their followers. Among these several key names, themselves psychiatrists, are to be found, including

Thomas Szasz who in *The Myth of Mental Illness* was opposed to use of compulsion to treat people who in his view were struggling with problems of everyday life rather than some mental illness; Ronald Laing who saw the family and family power struggles accounting for much of what we call schizophrenia; and more recently a movement called 'critical psychiatry'. Psychiatrist Duncan Double is one of a small number of professionals who look beyond conventional explanations and treatment of people who have mental health problems.

Why is it that a movement called critical psychiatry can find favour? The answer lies in part in the general need by the public and professionals alike to examine alternatives to conventional treatments of a range of health problems. The increased use of supplements to assist diet, the use of acupuncture and homeopathy all stand testimony to the general dissatisfaction with the increased technical and scientific focus of medicine in general and by inference psychiatry. They do not absolutely reject the use of medication but rather put medication into a range of treatments rather than, as it sometimes is seen, as the only treatment.

The fundamental tenet of critical psychiatry is to challenge the evidence base and in so doing inevitably to look at the psycho-social aspects of the service user's life. Phil Thomas, a consultant psychiatrist puts this over very succinctly on the critical psychiatry website **www.critpsynet.freeuk.com/**

> *Critical psychiatry is part academic, part practical. Theoretically it is influenced by critical philosophical and political theories, and it has three elements. It challenges the dominance of clinical neuroscience in psychiatry (but does not exclude it); it introduces a strong ethical perspective on psychiatric knowledge and practice; it politicises mental health issues. Critical psychiatry is deeply sceptical about the reductionist claims of neuroscience to explain psychosis and other forms of emotional distress. It follows that we are sceptical about the claims of the pharmaceutical industry for the role of psychotropic drugs in the 'treatment' of psychiatric conditions. Like other psychiatrists we use drugs, but we see them as having a minor role in the resolution of psychosis or depression. We attach greater importance to dealing with social factors, such as unemployment, bad housing, poverty, stigma and social isolation. Most people who use psychiatric services regard these factors as more important than drugs. We reject the medical model in psychiatry and prefer a social model, which we find more appropriate in a multi-cultural society characterised by deep inequalities.*

Double explains that the main aim of critical psychiatry is to develop a more open approach to psychiatry and that professionals like social workers need to remain sceptical about the claims that drug companies make for the efficacy of their products. This is not about ignoring the advances and assistance that medication has made but more about seeing this as only one component of the toolkit (*Critical Psychiatry*: *Limits of Madness,* 2006).

To work in a truly empowering way can run counter to the imposition of a biomedical regime in which it is possible to see control and restraint as dominant features rather than enabling and understanding. It is important to understand the cultural context in which service users experience mental health problems and the role that poverty, poor housing and oppression play in someone's mental health. This is where we need to examine alternative explanations such as the social model and the impact of neuroscience.

Neuroscience and mental health social work

For some time social work has had an uneasy relationship with pretty much anything to do with science. It is seductive to get into binary explanations of the world of mental health – seductive yet simplistic – and the more that I learn about neuroscience makes me re-evaluate this position. The idea that there are clinical or medicalised models and then there are social or environmental models is just too far from the emerging knowledge base to be true and sustainable. There are numerous reasons to rethink your understandings and this section will concentrate, if briefly, on two of them.

First we have experienced between 1990–99 the so-called 'decade of the brain', which stemmed from an initiative instigated by the then US president George W. Bush to promote the public's awareness of the importance of brain research and to create the environment in which major research initiatives would be developed. This has been followed up by President Obama through an initiative estimated to cost $300m over the next ten years and under the catchy name of Brain Research through Advancing Innovative Neurotechnologies (BRAIN). Now this is important, as up to the introduction of the 'decade of the brain' we knew that the most recent and powerful medications for mental illness were pretty effective for many people, what we didn't understand was why they worked. Or at least our understanding was at a rather primitive level, rather like we know if we put diesel in a car the engine will work but we really don't know what happens in the combustion process. We now know that if we are to reduce the impact and incidence of mental illness we need to learn about the origins of the illness itself and this is where neuroscience comes in.

We have for some time realised that the language of the brain is electricity and new research is expected to uncover the complex circuitry in our brains into a dynamic mapping or picture of how our brains work and the aim is that this will enable more targeted interventions to be made in areas such as Alzheimer's disease and schizophrenia. Whereas in the past we have tended to separate the mind from the brain, for example if someone has a stroke we see this as a physical interruption of their activity stemming directly from damage to their brain yet in depression we tend to see low mood as a feature of the mind and interaction with the environment.

Even at a rather basic level this doesn't make too much sense if you see that stroke victims can improve functioning and wellbeing by taking part in counselling and that now through brain imaging we can recognise that depression has altered some of the pathways inside the brain and that medication can help to reverse this or provide an interruption to some of the damaged pathways. In this way it looks more promising to connect ideas about how the brain works with those of the mind. The latest research projects are large scale and worth even in the UK tens of millions of pounds and included in aims are the examination of how the brain translates risk into symptoms of mental illness and the anticipated outcome is for there to be much better treatments.

Until the 'decade of the brain' initiative few believed that once adulthood had occurred that the brain could still change. One result of this was a fairly fixed viewpoint about the role that genetics and the environment separately had. We know that even when fully mature the brain has plasticity and can change and be changed. We know that the brain for example is very susceptible to environmental impacts of all sorts. We also are beginning to understand that mental illness may be understood as a faulty circuit in the brain. Which circuits, which pathways, are still open to investigation but the evidence is starting to amass and looks promising.

So can we adopt a positive and optimistic approach and if so what impact will this have on social work practice?

The social model

The social model fits well with the general holistic approach of social work and is the underlying rationale for mental health social work although it is by no means as influential as the medical model. Nevertheless there are numerous examples of practice where the social model underpins effective practice (Ramon, 2001; Tew, 2002).

There are several different perspectives even within this model:

- social causation;
- labelling;
- critical theory;
- social constructivism; and
- social realism.

Whereas the conventional medical approach puts illness down to genetics, viruses or some other biomedical cause, the social model looks at social and environmental causes. The implications of the medical model are that illness *is* a matter of bad luck and one that needs an individual reaction, whereas the social model highlights the social causes and hence invites social reaction. This latter approach brings into play issues of power, oppression and social exclusion (Tew, 2002).

Social causation

Social causation is a particular perspective that helps us to understand the interaction between social disadvantage and mental disorder. A psychiatric diagnosis is largely accepted and the interest of the sociologist is in the effect that societal inequalities and social exclusion have had on the person's mental health. Other variables such as gender, ethnicity and class can be incorporated into this explanatory model.

The concentration of people who are diagnosed as having schizophrenia in inner city areas is an interesting example of this perspective. For although it is a 'fact' that the incidence of schizophrenia in inner city areas is much higher than in the suburbs and that schizophrenia is predominantly a lower-class disorder, this is far from being a causal relationship.

ACTIVITY **2.2**

What factor do you think could explain the concentration of people with schizophrenia in inner city areas? Write down your ideas.

There are many possibilities but among those in the literature are:

- The drift theory, in which people who are long-term sufferers of schizophrenia migrate from rural areas into cities where they can blend in more easily and where services are more likely to be concentrated. People with schizophrenia from upper classes may find that the debilitating effect of this disorder results in their being unable to maintain their position in society and a downward drift into the lower classes occurs.

- Alternatively it could be that being in poverty in cities is harder and more alienating for people and that this could result in increased incidences of the disorder.

Labelling theory

Perhaps one of the most influential theories is labelling theory, which describes a process by which '**primary deviance**' occurs, such as strange behaviour, which continues to be interpreted as mental disorder or '**secondary deviance**'.

Primary deviance, or the initial concerning behaviour, may not always be recognised as a mental disorder as people often explain this initial deviance in terms of everyday behaviour. Thus the person with a drinking problem may be tolerated by their partner who has convinced themselves that their behaviour is just another way of letting off steam, or the more bizarre behaviour may be dismissed as humorous. Pilgrim and Rogers (1999) describe this as the 'clinical iceberg' (p.13) with many symptoms missed when doctors making diagnoses explain behaviours outside the norm for that person in terms of what should be, rather than what is, happening.

Secondary deviance occurs when the diagnosis is made and the person takes on, or is seen to have taken on, the deviant role. In the same way that in primary deviance some behaviour gets interpreted as 'usual' then some of the deviant behaviour also is seen as what is typical of a mentally disordered person. The sociologist Erving Goffman (1961) describes this as the making of a psychiatric patient and writes about the role that the hospital plays as a total institution.

Psycho-social causes of mental disorder

The early part of this chapter concentrated on the medical model in which work with service users is focused upon trying to identify the cause of the mental disorder in order that we can intervene to restore better mental health. We then briefly looked at the social model and now need to see how these two models can be applied to every-day practice. Most professionals accept that the most likely cause of mental disorder is a complex interaction between a range of factors and that we need to find a way of encompassing biological, psychological and social factors that may be present. Newton (1988) is one of many academics who have constructed models that not only help us to see possible causes, but also to identify what might be done with service users to improve their functioning.

A simplified version of these models is set out in Figure 2.2 and shows how factors can interact with each other to determine whether in any given circumstance a person will develop either good or poor mental health. These factors are:

- predisposing or vulnerability factors including genetic components and previous family or personal history of mental health problems;

- social causative factors including the importance of class, social exclusion and racism in reinforcing mental disorder;

- psychological factors including loss, threats, highly critical relationships, resilience to adverse events and the extent of social support networks that precipitate or trigger the onset of disorder.

It is important that you realise that these models are an oversimplification of complex situations and that different authors use different terminology. Nevertheless they at least provide an indication of where people might be vulnerable and offer the possibility of intervention to help strengthen the weak areas.

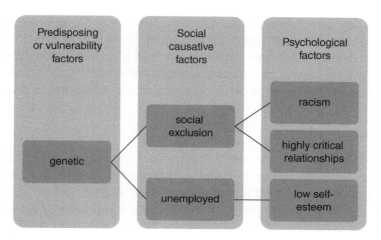

Figure 2.2   Psycho-social model

From Figure 2.2 you should be able to see how a number of variables can combine together to put someone in a very difficult mental state. You could substitute genetic with a family history of mental illness and similarly you could change other factors like unemployed with gender identity. The point is that this simple chart can help you to understand some of the processes that are often going on for people and crucially why it is that some people are much more vulnerable to mental illness than others. What might prevent the seesaw from tipping below might be the support of friends or the support of social work services.

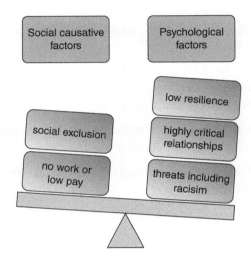

Figure 2.3   The tipping point?

This approach allows you to weigh up the factors and with the service user to work out what could be achieved to promote his/her mental good health. It also helps explain how people can face similar events but react differently. Thus although the service user may have a history of family mental health problems, he or she may be in a well-paid, satisfying job and with a network of social support. These factors could interact to provide protective rather than vulnerability factors. Of course the opposite might occur where no previous history of mental disorder is known but social exclusion and the resultant stress may increase the person's vulnerability to mental health problems.

Women and madness

My daughter is always keen to re-educate her father and recently lent me a book that is very relevant to this chapter. It is what you might call a classic as it was written in 1985 by Elaine Showalter titled *Women, Madness and English Culture, 1830–1980*. It is beautifully written and easy to read and what's more makes absolute sense. Her theme is that cultural ideas have shaped our views of what it is to be feminine and at the same time shaped the treatment and definition of mental disorder in women by giving it a sexual connotation. It is much more than that as she draws in vivid portraits of the men who have dominated psychiatry and the literature of writers like Doris Lessing and Mary

Wollstonecraft. This provides the reader with an alternative view of mental illness showing how in her view this is a consequence of, rather than a deviation of the traditional female role. It may be hard to get but if you can you will be rewarded!

Social work practice in a psycho-social context

The reality of intervening in people's lives is that you are working with something that is complex and multi-faceted (O'Sullivan, 1999). At the centre of our work is helping service users to manage their lives in ways that are better for them and for their families and society. Any intervention carries with it a degree of uncertainty about the effect that this intervention might have on the service user.

The present drive to integrate services for people with mental disorder in theory opens up the opportunity to provide a seamless service. Social workers will work alongside health colleagues and it will be obvious to both just what they each bring to the situation. The need for quality evidence on which to support the specific intervention is long overdue and the establishment of centres for evidence-based practice (Huxley, 2002, p.198) suggests that social care is beginning to embrace the idea of measuring changes that have occurred as a result of their and others' interventions.

The Cochrane Centre provides systematic reviews of the effects of health care interventions and has a number of mental health groups in the collaboration, all of which can be accessed through their website: **www.cochrane.org**. The evidence that we have already shows that psycho-social intervention can have a powerful effect on rehabilitation; respite care to relieve the impact on carers can delay hospitalisation; family interventions can alleviate some of the negative aspects of living with someone who has mental disorder; intervention aimed at improving the living environment and creating or supporting social networks is effective; family work can be effective in reducing the emotionally charged and overly critical family environments.

What works less well appears to be psychological debriefing after trauma, crisis intervention and case management (Huxley, 2002).

ACTIVITY 2.3

Examine Figure 2.2 and refer to either a case study that you know or one that is in this book. Lisa's story in Chapter 5 would work well for this activity.

Break down the case study into the factors that fit into this diagram and weight them according to your assessment of the likelihood of them increasing vulnerability or protecting against vulnerability to poor mental health.

You do not have enough detailed information to fully complete this task and that is perhaps the first important point to learn – analysis of causes is complex and requires careful collection of the 'evidence'.

The evidence that you have may well point to consideration of some of the factors such as does the service user belong to a black and minority ethnic group and if so is this likely to make them more vulnerable or less vulnerable? Similarly are they socially excluded? Is their financial situation stable?

If you work from right to left when looking at Figure 2.2 you should be able to get some idea of how various factors can interact to produce either a positive outcome or a negative one:

- **Predisposing or vulnerability factors** e.g. family with a history of mental disorder would make you more vulnerable to developing mental disorder.

- **Social causative factors** e.g. being unemployed or socially excluded (such as asylum seekers).

- **Psychological factors** e.g. no supportive relationships.

All of these factors could interact to produce low resilience, low self-esteem and therefore an increased likelihood of poor mental health.

You might want to think about what would have to change to increase resilience. A note of caution is needed, as it is unlikely that relationships between these factors would be simple or straightforward.

Stress is an intervening variable

Of course you probably realise that people experience similar events differently, the loss of job to one person could be a crushing blow that results in a vulnerability to depression yet to another it could be the very opportunity to go to college to get better qualified or to just take some time out. This will almost certainly be influenced by previous experience, family circumstances and financial position.

Epstein (1983) suggests that it is possible to learn better ways of coping with stress while writers like Cochrane (1983) point to the role that stress plays in pushing people either towards positive mental health or in the other direction. It is not just the experience of losing your job but the way in which this impacts upon you and, importantly, how you perceive the event. This approach does open up the prospect of working with the service user to recognise what makes them overstressed and to identify better ways to manage their stress. It is clearly not possible to reduce all the adverse events that affect a person's life but it is possible to get better at managing the situations that might cause them and their reactions to them.

EXAMPLE

Social workers working with families and young people who are on the road to recovery from an eating disorder can do work on some of the factors that cause the service user to feel under pressure about their eating habits. Among these short-term techniques are included:

- *not asking about what person has eaten;*

- *avoiding making comments about the food;*

- *not making comments about shape or size;*
- *not telling them that they look good or healthy;*
- *not making any comments about their weight.*

This puts the consideration of weight and size into the professional domain and removes everyday comments from family members that may be considered stressful.

Promoting mental wellbeing: a political approach

Newton provides information about what is needed to provide the necessary conditions to prevent mental disorder. Two possible approaches to prevention are either to work to reduce the vulnerability factors, or helping people to develop more positive responses and increased resilience to withstand stressful situations. It is a political approach as many of the social factors include the effects of social exclusion, racism and poverty.

Work that falls into the category of reducing vulnerability would include social workers being placed in schools and projects with specific funding, such as Sure Start. In both instances the work can be focused upon the young people and their families. Some of the work compensates for social disadvantage and could have a positive impact on mental health.

Promoting positive mental health: saving lives

In England it is estimated that one person kills himself or herself every two hours (HMG/DoH 2012). Although since a major government initiative in 2003 called the national Suicide Prevention Strategy incidence of suicide has been falling more remains to be done. The new strategy launched in 2012 builds upon this success and locates it within the government's overall mental health policy **No Health Without Mental Health** published in 2011. The implementation of this strategy is necessary to turn ambitious policy into reality. Some of the key factors that suggest some groups are more likely to commit suicide than others are described in the document.

It is hoped that by identifying key factors that are associated with suicide such deaths could be significantly reduced.

ACTIVITY **2.4**

Go back to Figure 2.2 and think where would be the best focus for a suicide prevention strategy. What factor would make people more vulnerable to suicide thoughts? Jot down your ideas.

(Continued)

(Continued)

COMMENT

You probably came up with most of the factors that are identified in the policy document. These would include people who are:

- *in low paid, unskilled work;*
- *unemployed;*
- *breaking up from their relationship;*
- *socially isolated;*
- *misusing drugs or alcohol;*
- *children and young people, especially those who are care leavers and those in the youth justice system;*
- *survivors of domestic abuse and violence including sexual abuse;*
- *lesbian, gay, bisexual and transgender people;*
- *Black, Asian and minority ethnic groups and asylum seekers.*

Having an impact in all these areas would help and we do not actually know which one would make the biggest difference. This requires a mixture of social policy and community initiatives.

Equally, working with service users who are depressed to improve their social networks would help, and so would encouraging service users to continue taking their medication.

Despite the methodological problems the government has moved forward with its intentions to affect the number of suicides with year-on-year reductions set as targets. Progress is being made but even so over 1,300 young adult men take their own lives each year in England, a number which has now overtaken road deaths as the biggest killer of young men in this age category (Brock and Griffiths, 2003). Overall over 4,200 people take their own lives each year. Some of the actions that have been taken include:

- reducing the pack sizes of aspirin and paracetamol in an attempt to make it more difficult for people to purchase large quantities of these tablets;
- improving the risk assessment on inpatient wards where acute patients are liable to be detained;
- establishing a research forum to improve the quality of the information that is available to professionals to ensure that professional practice is evidence based;
- working more closely with service user groups;
- setting up a number of pilot projects to target key at-risk groups such as young men.

With the last two actions social workers will be among the key professionals who will help to put these initiatives into operation.

It is too early to comment authoritatively about the effectiveness of this plan and authoritative evaluations are needed.

This chapter has introduced you to the two main theoretical approaches to understanding mental health. As required by the subject benchmark you should have developed your knowledge of the critical and research-based explanations that contribute to the knowledge base of social work, including the application to practice. As a social worker you need to have at least a basic understanding of the medical model and the major mental illnesses that can affect service users. You have also been introduced to the idea that in reality binary opposites such as a clinical or medical model and a social or critical seldom exist. This will enable you to have more meaningful dialogue with medical colleagues and to work in an informed way with service users.

Detail has been provided about mental disorder, intervention and treatment. Included in this has been a description of the main types of medication that are currently in use, and all this should help you to feel more confident and knowledgeable about mental health. The role of social workers in working with people who have mental disorder or mental health problems has been outlined and the provision of a schematic outline of psychosocial factors will help you to see where the best intervention ought to be made. As this model underpins most of social work practice when working with people who have mental health problems, it will be referred to over the next chapters.

In-depth case studies are provided in later chapters that build up your specific knowledge of depression, schizophrenia and eating disorders.

Stress busting tip

Preventing stress and promoting positive mental health by developing an effective support system

As you have seen in this chapter stress can play a large part in our mental health and can trigger mental health problems and disorder. Having a support system that provides support for you can help you and others to deal effectively and more healthily with stress. This support can be informal or formal, the key is what works for you. What does help is being able to talk things through with someone who helps you to see the positive side of things and can help you to construct solutions rather than dwelling upon the problems. This should help you to move into a 'glass half full' perspective rather than a 'glass half empty' one.

Consider your own support systems. If possible find a friend and go through this list recording your answers. The content of the discussion is confidential to you and you should only discuss what you feel comfortable with.

Support network

Do you currently have:

1. Someone on whom you can rely in a crisis?

2. Someone who makes you feel good about yourself?

3. Someone you can be totally yourself with?

4. Someone who will tell you, honestly, how well or badly you are doing?

5. Someone you can talk to if you are worried?

6. Someone who really makes you stop and think about what you are doing?

7. Someone who is lively to be with?

8. Someone who introduces you to new ideas, new interests, new people?

Of course to find all these 'ideal type' attributes in one person would be truly special and even if you did find such a person, putting all of this on them might be too much and put a strain on relationships. There are also key times when we may need extra support and have to either seek professional help or develop a new network.

If you have been able to reflect on this list you may now want to reflect a little more.

Is your support coming from one person? Is this from home or student life? Do you need a better balance between these two? What gaps have you got in your support network? What are you going to do about these gaps? If you have more gaps than you would like, work out how to alter this – you may want to find someone who can help you, perhaps a student counsellor.

FURTHER READING

Eldergill, A. (1997) seminal work *Mental Health Review Tribunals: Law and practice.* London: Sweet and Maxwell.

A classic in its own right and a surprisingly rich source for anyone who wants to read in depth on the origins, causes and treatment of mental disorder. In the 300 pages devoted to these topics he shows a remarkable grasp of detail and an enviable ability to explain these to non-medics. His work has greatly influenced the content of this chapter.

Montgomery, A. (2013) Toward the integration of neuroscience and clinical social work. *Journal of Social Work Practice: Psychotherapeutic Approaches in Health, Welfare and the Community,* 27: 3, 333–9.

One of the few reviews of social work and neuroscience that carves out a role for social work and highlights some of the reasons why this is resisted.

Pilgrim, D. and Rogers, A. (1999) *A Sociology of Mental Health and Illness* (2nd edition). Buckingham: Open University Press.

A best-selling text and one of a number of texts that illustrate the key perspectives on mental health. It has good chapters on social class inequalities and mental health, gender, race and ethnicity and age, all of which make for interesting and relevant reading.

WEBSITES

Social Trends can be downloaded free from **www.statistics.gov.uk**

Want to read more about neuroscience? This website is a good starting point: **www.dana.org/news/cerebrum**

Chapter 3

The policy and legal context for practice Part 1: history and new developments

Introduction: the need for legislation?

The end of law is, not to abolish or restrain, but to preserve and enlarge freedom.

(John Locke, 1690)

People who have mental health problems from time to time become vulnerable and a small but significant number may need treatment and care, even if this is against their wishes at the time. Such is the nature of mental disorder. Compulsory admission to hospital is just one part of the legislative framework but is so significant because of the potential infringement of the person's human rights. The implication for us as social workers is clear: if we are to be competent practitioners in mental health then we need to understand the relationship between the law and our practice and how to respond in different situations and to be able to work across organisations.

Just how much mental health law should be known by non-specialists is open to dispute but what is certain is that each and every one of us will work with people who have mental health problems and on occasion we will work with people who may be subject to some of the many parts of mental health legislation. Therefore it is important that all social workers, social care workers and nurses are familiar with the basic provisions of the law relating to mental health and some of the underlying tensions that exist in its execution, including the importance of ethics and values.

This chapter provides essential information about two important pieces of legislation, both amended in 2007 with most provisions in place by late 2008. Unlike previous chapters, there is only one case study, albeit a long one, for you to work through instead of smaller activities. Bear in mind that all law is experimental and subject to change and that there is no substitute for reading the actual statutes, codes of practice and regulations. Keeping up to date is essential not only to maintain your registration but also to ensure that you can engage with service users, carers and other professions in a manner, which exudes confidence that is founded on accurate information.

A very short history of mental health law

'Mad' people only became the concern of the public from about the middle of the eighteenth century, a point in history that coincides with the impact of modernism with the increased focus upon rationality and reason as characteristics of man (Shaw, 2007). Prior to this if you had mental health problems you were more likely to be kept within the family or to become one of the poor souls in the local workhouse. The perception that madness was the loss of reason and rationality resulted in a range of responses from locking people up to providing care and treatment.

During the early nineteenth century, county asylums developed with the aim of providing refuge and tranquility during which time residents would be able to recover their reason and rationality and be treated with respect. It was the job of magistrates to order admissions to such hospitals. At the same time private mad-houses flourished and soon thereafter concerns of abuse and ill-treatment were voiced, which resulted in the Madhouse Act of 1828. The continuing calls for regulation led to the 1845 Lunatics Act being passed by Parliament. At this time treatment was limited and the medical profession had little involvement and it was a while before madness became inextricably linked with the medical profession and the law. Locking people away in an asylum with various restraints became a familiar theme with the likes of Charles Dickens and other writers.

The growth in Europe of a treatment based upon the calm care for patients emerged in England at the York Retreat and was largely due to the influence of Tuke (1813) and earlier Pinel in France (1774). Through this approach it was expected that restraint could be replaced by helping people to regain their self-control of their madness.

Although the early reformers were enlightened social thinkers, it wasn't too long before the focus on 'moral treatment' once again gave way to a greater emphasis on the control of inmates' madness and the restriction of their liberty. The focus had again shifted to the need to 'protect the public' and in the 1890 Lunacy Act we witness the dominance of the legal profession and legal procedures over social reform and treatment.

This tension between treatment of the individual and the protection of the public can be seen to influence the development of our responses to mental health problems. First we move one way and then to another. In 1930 the Mental Treatment Act shifted the focus from custody and protection once again towards treatment and prevention. This reform was, according to some writers, a direct response to the emergence of treatments like insulin-coma therapy, electro-convulsive therapy and brain surgery (Shaw, 2007). This Act also introduced the first ideas about treating people in the community although it was many years before a significant move to the community actually occurred. Kathleen Jones, the first woman professor of social policy to be made a member of the Royal College of Psychiatry, describes the 1950s as a time when the three revolutions occurred (Jones, 1972). The first of these was the sudden advance in major medication and the arrival of anti-psychotics like chlorpromazine, which enabled the more florid symptoms in patients to be subdued; the second was the modernisation of hospitals and the increased range of facilities that were on offer; and the third revolution was the major legal reforms brought about in the 1959 Mental Health Act, principles of which still underpin modern-day legislation.

The move away from large asylums (psychiatric hospitals, as they were becoming known as) began to take hold in the late 1950s when two powerful forces happened to coincide. The first of these was largely a response to scandals about hospital care and a reaction to the reality that many patients on long-stay wards had become institutionalised and therefore unlikely ever to be able to leave the regime of institutional care. The second was the view, false as it proved to be, that care in the community would in fact be cheaper than keeping patients warehoused in expensive hospitals. Such tensions are still present today.

The 1983 Mental Health Act (MHA) was built upon the basic principles of the 1959 Act and even though the 2007 Act has made some significant changes the basic law remains. The 1983 Act saw the introduction of the approved social worker, who was a more skilled replacement for the 1959 mental welfare officer. It also introduced a strong legal framework and procedures in which any decision to admit someone to hospital had to be made. The influence of an American lawyer Larry Gostin, sometimes called the 'father of the Act', was evident with legalism embodied in this statute.

Calls for a more patient-centred and more imaginative legal framework gathered momentum from the late 1990s. At the same time public coverage of murders by ex-patients of mental hospitals meant that the government was anxious to put right as they saw it deficiencies in community care. One such murder was that by Christopher Clunis, who in 1992 stabbed Jonathan Zito, a complete stranger, in the eye, killing him. Jonathan, who had just arrived in the UK from Italy and was recently married, was waiting for an underground train with his brother at the time. Clunis was a well-known psychiatric patient, recently discharged, with a diagnosis of paranoid schizophrenia and a history of violence and non-compliance with treatment programmes. This resulted in calls for tighter surveillance and better resources for patients like Clunis to both protect them but also to protect the 'innocent' public.

Once again we can see tensions between the government's increased preoccupation with risk and control and the conforming to human rights legislation.

It was this preoccupation with managing risk and the new need to be compliant with human rights legislation, both hallmarks of a modernist agenda, that was to bring about confrontations between bodies like the Royal College of Psychiatry, the Mental Health Alliance and others to oppose many of the proposals by the government. The tension between personal freedom and protection of the general public had risen to the surface and was eventually to prevent the introduction of an entirely new law. The original reform process was initiated by the government in 1998, with a call for the most wide-ranging reform of mental health legislation since the 1950s. In 2002 and 2004, the government published proposals for new mental health legislation in England and Wales in the form of draft Mental Health Bills. However, faced with considerable opposition the proposals were abandoned in March 2006. In its place the government drafted a more streamlined proposal to amend the 1983 Act. The Bill was eventually introduced on 16 November 2006 and received Royal Assent on 19 July 2007. It reflects government concerns about managing risks and amends the Mental Capacity Act (MCA) by introducing deprivation of liberty safeguards (DoLS), which should comply with human rights legislation.

The large majority of people who have mental health problems do not need specialist treatment and even within this group there are many who can be treated in the community. Where hospital admission is indicated and they have capacity and the person is unwilling to go in, it must be that they have a mental disorder within the meaning of the Act that is of a nature or a degree that warrants detention and that this detention is necessary. The majority of admissions are through a civil process that does not involve courts but there are occasions when mentally disordered offenders may be detained in a psychiatric hospital or be transferred from prison to such a hospital.

However, not everyone is satisfied that the confrontational process that the government engaged with over reform has produced legislation that is in any way groundbreaking. In a press release the Mental Health Alliance claimed:

> We now have a Bill that for the first time gives people a right to an advocate when they are detained and that protects children from being put on adult wards inappropriately. We also have new safeguards over the use of electro-convulsive therapy, for people detained under the Mental Capacity Act, and for

the renewal of detention. These are hard-won improvements that are a credit to the persistence of activists from across the country.

But our members will be disappointed today that the Government has rejected changes to many other aspects of the Bill. It has failed to heed the evidence about the risks of significant over-use of community treatment orders and the excessive powers the Bill gives to clinicians. And it treats people with mental health problems as second-class citizens by allowing treatment to be imposed on those who are able to make rational decisions for themselves.

(Mental Health Alliance, July 2007 press release)

The legislation

The government changed the law about mental health after a lengthy period of debate and confrontation between a wide variety of interested parties and most of these provisions came into being by October 2008. The Mental Health Act 2007 amended the Mental Health Act 1983. This means that although the basic legislation remains the Mental Health Act 1983, we need to be familiar with the main provisions and amendments of this new legislation. This also introduces the deprivation of liberty safeguards (DoLS) – implemented in April 2009 – as an amendment to the Mental Capacity Act 2005. In a similar vein, the Domestic Violence, Crime and Victims Act 2004 was amended to increase the rights of the victims of crimes carried out by mentally disordered offenders.

There is a Mental Health Act Code of Practice that accompanies the Mental Health Act 2007 which, although not law, you must have regard to what it says, and if you deviate from this guidance you must be able to justify why. This chapter will examine some of main features of the Mental Health Act 2007 and the guidance contained within the Code of Practice.

The amendments to the legislation were carried out through a process of commencement orders that were made under the Mental Health Act 2007 and brought into force by the provisions of an amendment act, for example substituting references to 'an approved social worker' for those of 'an approved mental health professional'.

The Mental Capacity Act 2005 and the Mental Health Act 2007

Although every attempt has been made to guarantee accuracy, there is no substitute for going back to first principles and reading the Mental Health Act, the Mental Capacity Act and their associated Codes of Practice. The term 'patient' is used in the legislation, as is the male pronoun, and to avoid confusion these terms are used in this chapter. The detail of the MCA is covered in Chapter 4, Part 2.

Main purpose

The main reason for this new legislation is to provide a process by which a person with a mental disorder can be detained for treatment with or without his or her consent. It also provides legal processes that must be followed in order to safeguard the rights of the patient. The Department of Health overview states:

> *The main purpose of the legislation is to ensure that people with serious mental disorders which threaten their health or safety or the safety of the public can be treated irrespective of their consent where it is necessary to prevent them from harming themselves or others.*

(Department of Health guidance, 2007)

There are three ways in which a person may be admitted to a psychiatric hospital.

- Informally, which is often referred to as voluntary admission which is covered by s.131.
- Under the Deprivation of Liberty procedures in the amended Mental Capacity Act 2005.
- Compulsory detention under part 2 or part 3 of the MHA 1983.

Informal admission

If a person is capable of deciding whether to be admitted to hospital, he may be admitted with his consent. If he is refusing to consent he may not be admitted as an informal patient and the only option will be to detain him under the MHA 1983. An incapable patient may be admitted informally, but only if his care does not amount to a deprivation of liberty. An incapable patient may only be deprived of their liberty in accordance with new legal safeguards, referred to as deprivation of liberty safeguards (DoLS). (See Chapter 4.)

If a person with mental disorder needs to be admitted to hospital in the interests of his health or safety or for the protection of others and resists admission, then it is likely that they will be detained under the MHA 1983. If, however, he lacks capacity but is otherwise compliant with his treatment, his care will most likely be given under the MCA 2005.

There are circumstances where even if the patient agrees to go into hospital but is considered to be a danger to themselves or to others, that compulsory detention may be justified.

Principles underlying the MHA 1983 (and the MHA 2007 Amendment Act)

Unlike Scottish Mental Health legislation, which includes overt principles, the law for England does not and it is to the Code of Practice that we must look to find a statement of guiding principles, and these are set out below. These are essentially those that underpinned the 1959 MHA.

Purpose

Decisions under the Act should be taken with a view to minimising the harm done by mental disorder, by maximising the safety and well being (mental and physical) of patients and protecting them from harm.

Least restrictive alternative

Any intervention without the patient's consent must attempt to minimise the restrictions on the patient's liberty, having regard to the purpose for which they are imposed.

Respect

Diversity should be recognised and all workers should be aware of different cultures and how some behaviour may be misconstrued as mental disorder. The patient's wishes and feelings should be respected at all times and care should be taken to ensure that there is no unlawful discrimination.

Participation

Patients should be involved, as far as is practicable in the circumstances, in planning their own care and treatment to ensure that it is as effective and appropriate as possible. The involvement of carers, family members and others who have an interest in the patient's welfare must be encouraged (unless there are particular reasons to the contrary).

Resources

Decision-makers must seek to use whatever resources are available in an efficient, effective and equitable way. Decision-makers must take into account other people's perspectives on what is required.

The structure of the MHA 1983

The Act has ten parts and within these a variety of sections. Throughout this chapter you will see references to different parts of the Act. For example, you may find reference to Part 2 patients, who are people who have been made subject to some form of compulsory intervention under the Act in their own interests or to protect other people, without the involvement of the courts. They are also often known as 'civil patients'. Part 3 patients are those who have been made subject to a compulsory intervention under the Act by the courts, or who have been transferred to hospital from prison or another type of custody.

Definition of mental disorder (Section 1(2))

For the first time a single broad definition of mental disorder applies throughout the Act and the previous categories of mental illness, mental impairment, severe mental impairment and psychopathic disorder have been abolished. This broad definition will mean that patient need rather than a diagnostic label should determine whether compulsion is required.

Learning disability

The new legislation preserves the effect of the Act as it applies to learning disability. The effect of abolishing the four categories of mental disorder will be that all the powers in the Act will in future apply to all types of mental disorder. There is a special provision which means that (as now) learning disability will only be treated as a mental disorder for those purposes if it is associated with abnormally aggressive or seriously irresponsible conduct on the part of the person concerned.

Powers to detain and treat people without their consent

As a social worker you are far more likely to come across people who have mental health problems and are receiving treatment (if any) in the community or who are in hospital on a voluntary or informal basis. However, the removal in certain circumstances of a patient's liberty is so serious that you need to understand both the process and the role of the various people who implement the appropriate sections of the legislation.

Article 5 of the European Convention on Human Rights protects patients against arbitrary detention and because of the seriousness of compulsory detention three safeguards exist.

- Except in an emergency the person must have a mental disorder that has been established on the basis of objective medical expertise.

- The mental disorder must warrant detention.

- Detention must continue only while the mental disorder persists. Therefore those carrying out the detention must review the situation at regular intervals to ensure that the criteria continue to be met.

With the above criteria in mind, it should be obvious that there needs to be a clear process to compulsorily admit someone to hospital. There are professionals who perform key tasks in the legislation, but first let us examine just who the major parties are.

Professionals and others concerned with the operation of the Act

The present legislation has broadened the group of professionals and others who can be involved in the operation of the Act. These are the Approved Mental Health Professional (AMHP), who replaces the former ASW and is the professional who applies for admission; the Approved Clinician (AC), who is a mental health practitioner – not restricted to just doctors – who for the purposes of the Act can make certain decisions about medical treatment that can be given without patient's consent. Significantly, only approved clinicians can go on to be Responsible Clinicians (RC), who replace the Responsible Medical Officer (RMO) and who has the lead clinical responsibility for detained patients. The nearest relative is continued and can play an important part.

There are increased opportunities for social workers to become involved in a range of mental health work and even in the complex world of legislation social workers will be using their skills to communicate with people, helping them to understand the challenges and problems they face and providing statutory bodies with reports and assessments.

What is an AMHP?

An AMHP or Approved Mental Health Professional is the replacement for the ASW or Approved Social Worker. The role is now opened up to other professionals who have a range of experiences and skills in mental health including nurses, psychologists and occupational therapists and of course social workers but not doctors. It remains to be seen how effective this is and it does offer a different skill mix and a range of experiences. Arrangements for approvals are set out in the Mental Health (Approval of Persons to be Approved Mental Health Professionals) (England) Regulations 2008 ('the AMHP regulations').

AMHPs can be employed by local social services authorities (LSSAs) but could also be employed by NHS trusts or even be self-employed. Irrespective of their status the AMHP will be appointed to the role by an LSSA. He must exercise independent judgement and be personally accountable for his own practice and need not follow any directions that might be given to him by the LSSA.

Existing Approved Social Workers (ASWs) became AMHPs overnight when the Act came into force in 2008. LSSAs in conjunction with many universities are offering updating courses that will help prepare the newly converted AMHP for their role.

Why have an AMHP?

It is a legal requirement that the Local Social Services Authority (section 114 amended) appoint AMHPs who have an appropriate level of competence. AMHP functions include making applications for admission to hospital and guardianship applications, and agreeing that patients should become supervised community treatment patients (SCT).The AMHP is pivotal to the admissions process and provides an important counterbalance to a more medicalised view of the individual's circumstances.

The AMHP is expected to:

- bring to any decision a separate perspective and model of mental health;
- provide a detailed and comprehensive understanding of social care and community resources;
- be able to assess social factors that provide the context in which the 'patient' is being seen;
- be able to carry out a comprehensive risk assessment;
- be trained to explore the least restrictive alternatives to any hospital admission;

- make the application to detain a patient founded on the recommendation of the doctor or doctors;

- organise and manage the practical aspects of assessments and, if necessary, admissions to hospital.

Use of the Act

The number of people who are being made the subject of a compulsory admission order under the Mental Health Act continues to rise. In the annual report from the CQC they report that there was 48,631 detentions in England of men and women in hospital for assessment and/or treatment during 2011/12. A further 4,220 people were made subject to a community treatment order (CTO). They report that this is an increase of 5% in hospital detentions and a 10% increase in the use of CTOs compared to the previous year (CQC Monitoring the MHA 2011/12). Across this year there appears to be a decrease in the number of people admitted informally or voluntarily.

Table 3.1   Detentions: admission patterns all hospitals under the MHA by reporting year

Year of admission	2008–9	2009–10	2010–11	2011–12	2012–13
On admission to hospital	27,946	30,187	29,557	30,900	32,224
Subsequent to admission	14,701	13,712	13,397	13,680	14,249
Following use of s.136	1,753	1,922	2,376	2,582	2,426
Following revocation of CTO	143	779	1,018	1,469	1,509
Total all detentions	44,543	46,600	46,348	48,631	50,408

(Source: KP90, Health and Social Care Information centre)

Table 3.2   The use of Part II and Part III admissions by year

Year of admission	2008–9	2009–10	2010–11	2011–12	2012–13
Total admission	27,946	30,187	29,557	30,900	32,224
Part II section 2	16,153	18,385	19,163	20,931	22,477
Part II section 3	9,601	9,545	8,174	7,701	7,776
Part III	2,138	2,191	2,138	2,130	1,788
Other Acts	54	66	82	138	183

Table 3.2 shows that across all years Part II accounts for the majority of admissions to hospital and within that section 2 (admission for assessment and to provide treatment if necessary) has been used to an increasing extent. This rise in the use of section 2 over the recent years may explain the reduction in section 3 admissions which in turn might reflect earlier intervention on the part of community teams. It may also be in part explained by the reluctance of some hospitals to accept informal patients.

Part III of the MHA relates to people who are admitted as a result of criminal proceedings, they can of course be accused, convicted and awaiting trial or conviction.

Contrastingly, the use of short-term sections such as s.5 have declined by about 14 % over the last two years and show a steady decline during the overall reporting period.

Nearest relative (NR)

This is an important role and safeguard under the MHA even though there has been considerable discussion as to whether this role should continue. The NR has a range of functions in relation to patients who may be detained or liable to be detained under Part 2 of the MHA. These include the right to apply for compulsory admission or guardianship; be consulted before any application is made by an AMHP; within certain parameters object and stop any application for detention or guardianship; discharge the patient; apply to the Mental Health Tribunal for discharge; and receive information about the patient's and their own rights under the MHA.

Who is the NR is determined according to a list, which begins with husband, wife or civil partner, father then mother, etc. Amendments to the MHA 1983 made by MHA 2007 ensure that in the case of civil partners, one will be the NR of the other, regardless of the length of their cohabitation (and even if they don't cohabit at all). Where there is more than one 'relative' it is the oldest who comes first. The nearest relative of a 'looked after child' is generally the local authority.

It is possible for a NR to be displaced and this process involves application to the County Court (s.29). The AMHP may bring forward such an application and if successful it will be the local authority that is appointed as a NR. It is possible for a patient to make such an application and for a displacement order to be made on an additional ground; that the NR is not a suitable person to act as a NR.

Offences

Part 9 of the MHA identifies additional safeguards that were created to protect vulnerable individuals at the time when they are suffering with a mental disorder. This also means that failure to act appropriately could result in health and social care professionals facing civil or criminal proceedings if the quality of care and treatment falls short.

Independent Mental Health Advocates (IMHAs)

From November 2008 in Wales and April 2009 in England a new role of Independent Mental Health Advocate was introduced and is available for most patients who are detained for treatment and those who are subject to guardianship or supervised community treatment. This service is still developing and at present provision is rather variable. There is a danger than this will stay at a 'by request' programme and the opportunities for a proactive service in which IMHAs advertise and promote services slip by. There is a similar role under the Mental Capacity Act called IMCA (covered in Chapter 4).

It would be easy to confuse the IMCAs with IMHAs but careful consideration to the respective roles reveals little overlap between the two. For the most part, patients who have an IMHA will not be eligible for an IMCA. If a qualifying patient requests it, the advocate can meet with not only the patient but also his or her nearest relative, responsible clinician or an AMHP. The patient's advocate will – if the patient consents – have the right to see any hospital or local authority records relating to the patient. Importantly the advocate can meet with the patient in private and visit anyone who is professionally concerned with the patient's treatment. The advocate will also have the right to meet the patient in private, and to visit and interview anyone professionally concerned with the patient's medical treatment.

Approved Clinician (AC)

This is an important new role that is not restricted to doctors and could include social workers. Prior to the 2007 Act this was restricted to consultant psychiatrists. The role gives powers to detain inpatients for up to 72 hours (see s.5) in addition to the registered medical practitioner if the AC believes that an application for admission to hospital should be made. The AC may visit and assess patients at the request of the patient's nearest relative for a range of reasons including advice about powers of discharge or referral. The AC is expected to be competent to carry out assessments about the presence of and the nature of mental disorder, to be able to lead a multidisciplinary team and to be able to understand different treatment modalities and their applicability to a range of patients.

In an 18-month pilot scheme a social worker is to take on this senior role and oversee the care delivered to people on community treatment orders in the Norfolk and Suffolk Mental Health Trust. This is the first time that a social worker has taken on this role and if the evaluation shows it is a success it will open up opportunities for social workers and improve prospects for innovative treatments for patients (*Community Care*, 27 November 2013). A non-medical AC will not be able to prescribe medication for a patient which opens up the prospect of overlap and disagreements between the AC and the prescriber.

Responsible Clinician (RC)

This is the professional who has overall responsibility for decisions about the treatment of detained patients, a role that was formerly carried out by the Responsible Medical Officer (RMO), who was of course a doctor. However, the new role of responsible clinician need not be filled by a doctor and could be a nurse, psychologist, an occupational therapist or a social worker, providing that they have undergone the appropriate specialist training. Before becoming a responsible clinician all professionals will need to have been an approved clinician. This is expected to be seen by these listed professionals as a career path position. This is an important change as for the first time in recent history the treatment and detention of patients lie in the hands of a range of professionals including but not limited to the medical profession.

The responsible clinician (RC) is defined in s.34 of the MHA 1983 as amended by MHA 2007.

Section 12 approved doctors

A section 12 doctor is a medical practitioner who has been approved under this section as a practitioner who has special interest and expertise in the diagnosis and treatment of mental disorder. Most family doctors do not have this level of understanding and experience and will be required to undertake specialist training before they can be appointed as a section 12 doctor.

Hospital managers

The hospital managers are by law the body responsible for detaining a patient under the MHA 1983. In a NHS hospital, the managers will be the NHS trust responsible for the hospital, and in an independent hospital it will be the person registered in respect of that hospital. They must oversee the detaining documents to ensure that their treatment and care is in accord with the provisions of the specific section under which the patient is detained. They must also ensure that the patient has been informed of their rights and that as far as possible the patient understands such rights (with clear implications for people who cannot see, hear or for whom English is not a comprehensible language).

Admission to hospital (compulsory detention)

As a social worker you need to understand what happens to patients when they are detained in hospital, what to advise their carers and what they should expect from the hospital and community services. Having described the key people concerned with the compulsory detention of patients, it is now necessary to see what part they play in such a decision. Basically in every compulsory 'civil' admission process the AMHP or the nearest relative makes the application on the prescribed form (which is a statutory form), which is founded upon at least one medical recommendation. Neither party on their own can admit a patient to hospital. To help to make this clearer, let us identify some key decision-making points.

- Does the patient have the capacity to make a judgement about their condition?

- If the answer to the above is no, are they resisting going into hospital?

- If the answer is that they do have capacity to make their own decisions, are they willing to go into hospital on their own volition?

- If they are not willing to go into hospital, are the circumstances such that they will meet legal criteria that will permit compulsory admission?

- If the answer is no, then no admission will occur but community services and support should be mobilised.

- If the answer is that the patient does meet the criteria for compulsory admission, is this a situation which would be classed as an emergency?

- If the patient meets the criteria for admission, do we know what the nature and extent of the mental disorder are or do we need an assessment to be carried out?

- If the patient meets the criteria for admission and we know the nature and extent of the mental disorder, is there treatment available at the hospital?

This is complex, as the deprivation of anyone's human rights as a compulsory detention should be a last resort and in line with the principles that underpin the legislation. The following case study should help to understand how such questions are addressed.

The AMHP role in practice

There are a number of statutory duties placed specifically on the shoulders of an AMHP by the Mental Health Act. An important function is under s.13 and that is to decide whether to make an application for compulsory admission to hospital under Part 2 of the Act (Brown et al., 2009, p.29). The AMHP is usually the professional who will make the application although it can legally be the NR in which case the AMHP will assist the NR. A key framework for the admission decision is the Code of Practice (DoH, 2009). This provides guidance as to how the Act should be implemented and includes some useful discussion about underlying principles. The Code does not have the force of law but should only be departed from where there are cogent reasons (*Munjaz v Mersey Care NHS Trust (2005)*).

The assessment process should never be considered as a straightforward form filling exercise and should instead be approached with a degree of criticality and questioning of the evidence. Gathering information to help better understand a person's situation is never easy especially when that person may well be under a great deal of stress, Nevertheless this should be done in a manner that respects the service user's dignity and preserves as far as practical their confidentiality. This is known as utilising emotional labour, which in summary is the ability on the part of the professional to manage the stressful aspects of the work, often at their height during the assessment phase, and still act in a professional way suppressing to a large extent one's own feelings.

CASE STUDY

This is a long case study that if you work through will help you to understand the process that lies behind Part 2 admissions or civil admissions.

There is a summary table shortly after this case study (Table 3.3) that shows the differences between the main sections of the Act under Part 2.

Susan is a 17 year old about whom her parents have become increasingly concerned. She has been acting strangely by staying up all night and sleeping throughout the day. This has gone on for a couple of weeks and there has been a marked deterioration in her behaviour since she last saw her family GP, who had prescribed her some antidepressants. The family were struggling to cope with this behaviour but now had found some notes that they took as intent to seriously harm herself. She flew into a rage when she discovered that they had been in her room reading her notes and opening up her emails on her computer.

The doctor has now arrived and Susan has shut herself in her room and is screaming and throwing stuff around the room. She is shouting abuse and threatening to kill herself if anyone comes near her. The doctor is confused as to what to do next but thinks admission to the local psychiatric unit would be appropriate.

What is the next step?

This is a tricky situation but let us work through the key decision points mentioned earlier.

First, does she have capacity? By all accounts, when she is calmer she is perfectly capable of understanding information that is related to the decision about her situation and would be able to retain this information and to weigh up the alternatives. In other words, she would almost certainly be deemed to be able to make a decision about whether she should go into hospital, and therefore is not an incapable person within the meaning of the MCA. The result of this is that the initial decision to use either the MHA or the MCA is now firmly on the side of using the MHA.

Is Susan resisting going to hospital? This is difficult to say as she is in such a state that communication is difficult, but as far as the doctor can determine she will not go anywhere, let alone a hospital.

Next, does she have a mental disorder of a nature or degree that warrants detention in hospital for at least a limited period? Her family GP has of course been treating her for depression and has prescribed a course of antidepressants. Does this mean that she has a mental disorder that is so serious as to warrant detention in hospital? It does not if this was the only evidence but the latest outburst and the worsening of her behaviour may indicate that she might meet the criteria. Let's suppose that on balance the GP thinks she does meet the criteria for a mental disorder. This alone is not enough. Susan must now meet the grounds that she ought to be detained in the interests of her own health or safety or with a view to the protection of others. This too is a judgement call and if this ground or condition is not met, no admission can proceed against her wishes.

Is the situation a genuine emergency? This is important because in an emergency a patient may be admitted to hospital on the basis of a single medical recommendation providing that the applicant (either the AMHP or the NR) agrees. If it would cause 'undesirable delay' to wait for a second recommendation, section 4 allows the patient to be detained for up to 72 hours while that recommendation is sought. Remember that most family GPs are not mental health specialists. If, within the 72-hour period, a second medical recommendation is obtained, the patient will be deemed to be detained under section 2 (and to have been so from the point at which they were first admitted under section 4). If this situation can wait (there are time limits) the doctor needs to decide to use either a section 2 or a section 3 admission.

Let us assume that the doctor decides that although in his view an admission is necessary, he thinks it better and more appropriate for this to be a section 2, which is for assessment followed by treatment if necessary. His justification would be that as no one knows what the nature of the mental disorder is, an assessment is needed and at this stage the exact nature of any treatment is unknown. The existing antidepressant medication appears ineffective. If Susan is to be admitted under section 2, the two doctors need to make their recommendation and either the AMHP or the NR needs to make the actual application.

It is likely that the applicant will be the AMHP rather than the NR and many professionals think that this would be more appropriate given that at some point Susan will return back to the family. The AMHP plays a key role as they will be the applicant and without them no admission will occur. The AMHP has an independent decision to make and they are required to consider the relative merits of admission taking into account the principle of the 'least restrictive alternative'. The AMHP must also take into account the views of the NR about admission and if the AMHP decides not to go ahead they must explain to the NR in writing why they have made this decision and what the alternatives proposed are.

If the application goes ahead the AMHP must arrange and co-ordinate the assessment and this will include the arrangements to take Susan to the hospital. The Code of Practice is clear that although AMHPs act as independent professionals they must exercise their judgement based on the evidence that is available and to take into account the availability of community alternatives (DoH, Mental Health Act 1983, draft Revised Code of Practice (2007) Para 4.4).

How does the AMHP make this assessment? It is the duty of the AMHP to interview the patient in a *suitable manner* and to satisfy him or herself that *in all the circumstances of the case it is the most appropriate way of providing the care and treatment,* which Susan needs. But how does he achieve this when Susan has shut herself in her room and is screaming and shouting? This is where the experience and the skill of the AMHP will come into play to try to get to interview Susan. Carrying out an interview through a closed door would not be considered as a suitable manner. Let us assume that through a combination of persistence and skill the AMHP has interviewed Susan and she remains agitated and still threatening to self-harm. Two doctors have seen her, including a section 12 approved one, and they are recommending admission to hospital.

CASE STUDY Continued

The AMHP has now completed the application process founded on the two doctors' recommendations and now the ambulance has arrived to convey Susan to hospital.

What happens next?

Applicants for compulsory admission under Part 2, irrespective of who is the applicant, are authorised by s.6(1) to take and convey or to authorise others to so do. In this case the AMHP has authorised the ambulance staff to carry out this responsibility. The use of an ambulance is preferable to other forms of transport. While they are doing this they have the power of a constable including arresting any person who is wilfully obstructing them. The conveyance to hospital has to be lawful and humane and if the patient is likely to be troublesome the AMHP should give advice and assistance. Many areas have a joint policy that puts limits on the length of time that should elapse between a first call for an ambulance and the arrival time. In many areas this is 2 hours but you might find it helpful to check just what this is in your area.

In the unlikely event of Susan escaping, the person who had the patient in legal custody has the power under s.18 to retake them into custody with a view to satisfactorily conveying them to hospital.

CASE STUDY *Continued*

Susan has now arrived at the hospital. What should happen next?

It is important to note that a child is defined as anyone who is under 18 years old. There is no age limit for the application of the MHA although guardianship cannot be used where the patient is under 16. There is a legal duty to provide suitable age-related accommodation under s.31 of the MHA; therefore Susan should not be admitted to an adult ward. In cases where a child or adolescent is concerned, at least one of the applicants or doctors should have specialist child or adolescent knowledge.

Applications for compulsory admission are addressed to the hospital manager and it therefore falls to them to ensure that the grounds for admission are valid and that all the paperwork is complete. In addition there is a quality-assurance role in that periodically all documents must be audited and those responsible must be aware of the sorts of errors that are able to be rectified and those that cannot be changed. The hospital manager also has the legal responsibility to inform patients of their right to advocacy and their rights to appeal to the mental health review tribunal where this is relevant. In some cases, information must also be provided to the patient's NR. These steps must be taken as soon as practicable after admission and should be repeated if there is any doubt that the patient has fully comprehended the information.

If Susan's NR had made the application (her father?) then the hospital manager is required to let the LSSA know as soon as practicable. Once this information is

Table 3.3 *The compulsory admission process to hospital: Summary of main provisions*

	Section 2 (assessment)	Section 3 (treatment)	Section 4 (emergency)
What is it?	Provides for admission for those who have a mental disorder that warrants detention. Interests of their health or safety or protection of others	For those who are suffering from a mental disorder and it is necessary for their health or safety or for the protection of others and that this cannot be provided without detention and that the appropriate treatment is available	To be used only in an emergency and where unnecessary delay would be caused by waiting for a second medical recommendation
What is the effect?	Length of detention is up to 28 days and cannot be extended	Up to six months initially and can be renewed for a further six, then in periods of one year	Up to 72 hours. Can be converted to s.2 providing second doctor recommends and applicant agrees
Process	NR or AMHP is the applicant. Plus two doctors, one of whom must be s.12 approved	NR or AMHP is the applicant. Plus two doctors, one of whom must be s.12 approved	NR or AMHP plus one doctor who ideally should know the patient and should only be used where it is an emergency
Notes	This is the section by which those whose mental disorder is uncertain would be admitted under	This is the 'main' section by which patients are admitted to hospital to have treatment	With this section the patient is deprived of a fundamental safeguard in that the doctor who recommends need not have specialist mental health knowledge

received the LSSA will direct an AMHP to visit and prepare a social circumstances report, which is forwarded to the managers.

Having worked through a section 2 admission you should by now have got the general idea about the legal process of admission and some of the issues that may arise during such processes. The next step is to look at some of the other more commonly used parts of the legislation, which are all variants of the section 2 admission process. These are summarised in Table 3.3.

Applications for admission for assessment or treatment may be made for patients who are already in hospital.

Holding powers pending applications in respect of patients already in hospital (sections 5(2) and 5(4))

In certain circumstances, informal inpatients may be detained temporarily in the hospital pending the making of an application, as described below. This does not apply to patients who are already detained on the basis of an application under the Act, or to SCT patients. There are two main powers; one for doctors and the other for certain prescribed nurses.

Holding power of doctor or approved clinician in charge of patient's treatment (s.5 (2))
Inpatients can be detained in a hospital for up to 72 hours if the doctor or approved clinician in charge of their treatment reports that an application for admission under sections 2 or 3 ought to be made.

Nurses' six-hour holding power (s.5 (4))
Nurses 'of the prescribed class' may authorise the detention for up to six hours of a patient who is already being treated for mental disorder in the hospital as an inpatient if they think that:

- The patient is suffering from mental disorder to such a degree that it is necessary for the patient's health or safety or for the protection of others, for the patient to be immediately restrained from leaving the hospital; and it is not practicable to secure the immediate attendance of a doctor or an approved clinician.

Compulsory powers in the community
Community treatment orders – section 17A

When the new law came into being one of the more controversial features was the introduction of compulsory supervision in the community (often referred to as supervised community treatment or SCT). These measures had been long sought after by some professionals most notably psychiatrists and at the outset the government seemed determined that this should in effect be the flagship of the reforms to the mental health legislation. Their view was that the present law provided little for those service users who had long-term and enduring mental health problems. There was a view that readmissions to hospital were often as a consequence of patients not taking their pre-scribed medication. The result was that for many patients admissions and discharge from hospital became something of a 'revolving door'. One solution was to introduce some form of measure that would compel discharged patients to take medication.

This was met with resistance from a coalition of professionals who were equally strongly opposed to these measures. At first glance they appear to be a necessary response to the reduction in inpatients' facilities following widespread deinstitution-alisation even though at the time of implementation their efficacy was unproven.

Since the closure of many large-scale psychiatric hospitals patients with psychosis are treated routinely in the community. Many are subject to what is often referred to as the 'revolving door syndrome' by which they often experience repeated readmission.

Supervised community treatment orders (CTOs) were introduced on November 2008 in England and Wales. The main aim of such orders was to enable patients who were under this power to be monitored clinically and to permit recall for assessment if it thought that their situation was deteriorating or for example the patient was refus-ing to take medication. Interestingly and worthy of note is that these orders do not permit medication to be administered against the patient's will and therefore if this is considered necessary recall to hospital is the only way that this can happen.

To be eligible for a CTO a patient must be liable to be detained under s.3 of Part 2 or a hospital order or a transfer direction under Part 3 of the Act and who, without contin-ued treatment, is assessed as being a risk to their own health or safety or to the health and safety of others. A CTO will be imposed when a responsible clinician (usually a consultant psychiatrist) and an approved mental health practitioner (usually a social worker) both agree that the patient needs supervision following on from detention in hospital and that without this supervision they would be likely to relapse and have to be readmitted to hospital under a compulsory admission. The CTO is made for an initial six months, renewable for a further six months and thereafter in one-year terms.

Making a CTO is a lengthy process during which the AMHP is expected to discuss with all relevant parties the effect of the CTO and to take note of any objections or potential risks that are raised. This may take several days to achieve but of course the patient is already in hospital so this is routine rather than emergency. There are, however, concerns that the gap between the RC completing the initial form and the AMHP agreeing can extend to the point where it might be questionable if the applica-tion is still current. The CTO will usually have conditions, such as where the patient can live, attendance at regular assessments and often includes that the patient takes prescribed medication, but if the patient subsequently refuses their medication this cannot be administered by force and a recall for up to 72 hours can be achieved with-out a formal readmissions process.

The concept

Fennel suggests that there are disturbing features of CTOs from a human rights perspective as the conditions and restrictions on personal freedom are left to the professional discretion of the health professionals (Fennel, 2007, p.212). According to the CQC a number of patients are worried that it isn't clear to them when the CTO will have served its purpose and a full discharge can be made (CQC, 2013, p.77). Against this some patients are content to be on a CTO because it gives them access to the sorts of services that they feel they need. In order for the CTO to be effective there needs to be good channels of communication between the service user and the professionals who are 'supervising' although evidence suggests that this is not always the case.

Use of CTOs

Since their introduction in November 2008 the annual use has increased steadily and on March 2013 there were 5,218 people subject to a CTO with 4,647 CTOs actually made during 2012/13, an increase of 10% over the previous year (hscic, October 2013). There is however considerable variation in the use of CTOs by providers with one area scarcely using them and another seeing 45% of discharges from section 3 to the CTO. We can only speculate about why this is and further research is needed before any judgement can be made.

The evidence

When CTOs were introduced I wrote that this was a leap into the unknown. This was in spite of similar orders having been introduced in North America and Australasia (edition 4, p.64). At that time the largest randomised trial of CTOs had just been funded with the University of Oxford taking the lead. Now in 2013 the initial findings of this huge study are known and similar to two previous studies and somewhat surprisingly,

> ...they did not find any evidence that CTOs achieve their purpose of reducing readmission in so-called revolving door patients with a diagnosis of psychosis. The evidence is now strong that the use of CTOs does not confer early patient benefits despite substantial curtailment of individual freedoms

> (*Lancet*, vol. 381, published online 26 March 2013)

The question that you might want to address is whether the infringement of patient rights justifies the use of CTOs. Some critical commentators refer disparagingly to CTOs as 'psychiatric ASBOS' – perhaps a good topic for a dissertation or long essay?

Service user views

One of the most common concerns raised by service users was 'poor interaction' as they saw it between themselves and community staff. In some cases this was compounded by the absences of an effective care plan (CQC, 2013, p.79). Infrequent and unplanned contact could result in the service user feeling that this order was really about keeping them medicated rather than about making progress with recovery. The reorganisation in many areas of mental health services has added to the difficulties with the responsibility for the patient transferring from the hospital team to a community team bringing with it the prospect for the patient to form new relationships.

Leave of absence (s.17)

Section 17 leave was originally intended as a measure that would allow detained patients to go home for short periods or to go out to shops nearby to the hospital to help determine if they were ready to be discharged from hospital. However, no restrictions were made on the length of this leave. With the arrival of the CTO this should replace the longer-term uses of s.17 leave. Indeed, where an RC is proposing to give a detained patient leave of seven days' duration or more, he may do so only if he has first considered imposing a CTO on the patient.

Responsible after-care bodies (s.117 (3))

The duty to provide after-care services under section 117 stands by itself. It is not a duty to provide services under other legislation (e.g. the National Assistance Act 1948 or the NHS Act 2006). As a result, normal rules about commissioning responsibility (in the NHS) or ordinary residence (for social services) do not apply. The consequence of this is that the responsible after-care bodies are the LSSA and the PCT for the area in which the person concerned is resident or is sent on discharge by the hospital in which the patient was detained.

Guardianship

Guardianship orders can be either a civil process (Part 2) or can be made through the courts (Part 3). The consequences of a guardianship order are set out in Table 3.4. The main provision is that guardianship may be used to restrict patients' liberty (e.g. by determining where they are to live) but it may not be used to deprive them of their liberty (i.e. to detain them).

If the patient lacks the capacity to make a decision for themselves and their best interests would be to reside in a hospital or care home, and to be deprived of liberty there, it may be necessary to use the DoLS procedure in order to obtain an appropriate authorisation under the MCA. If such patients require treatment for mental disorder in hospital and they object to being admitted, it might be necessary to admit (or transfer) them to hospital under the MHA.

Part 2 Civil orders

Although this has not been used anything like the extent to which it was envisaged, it remains a less restrictive alternative to hospital detention. The range of patients eligible has been extended and with powers generally contained in Part 2 of the Act it is expected that more orders will be made. Either the AMHP or the nearest relative can apply to have a person made subject to a guardianship order. The patient must have a mental disorder of a nature or degree that warrants guardianship and it must be in the interests of the patient's welfare or for the protection of others.

Part 3 Court-made orders

The offender being considered for guardianship must be over 16 years of age and have a mental disorder of a nature or degree that warrants guardianship. The court

Table 3.4   Summary of main compulsory powers in the community

	Section 117	Section 17	SCT or CTO	Section 7 Guardianship
What is it?	Places a duty on the PCT and LSSA to provide aftercare for patients who have been detained on any order specifying treatment, e.g. s.3 or s.37	Enables the RC to grant leave for a detained patient to reside in the community, during which time the patient agrees to treatment that can include taking medication as a condition for discharge. Failure to comply can result in readmission to hospital	Eligible patients are those who are liable to be detained in a hospital or if a Part 3 patient be subject to a hospital order. A patient on this order will be known as a community patient. The treatment must be available in the community and it must be necessary for the patient's health or safety or for the protection of others that he receives this treatment	An order that is less restrictive than being detained in hospital while retaining the same powers under Part 2. Patients must be over 16 years of age. It was thought that this section would herald a move towards more care in the community but the small number of orders actually made suggest otherwise.
What is the effect?	Imposes a duty on the local authority to assess a patient for eligibility for community services	Although the patient must agree to treatment in the community there is no provision whereby the patient can be made to accept treatment including medication	Patient must reside at an agreed address, be available for treatment and receive it. Patient must abstain from particular behaviours. Note the obligation to receive medical treatment, which is stronger than in s.17	Three powers are conferred on the guardian (s.8). The patient must reside at an agreed address; attend for treatment; and allow access to address of certain specified persons. Where the court makes the order it in effect assumes the role of the applicant.
The process	The duty applies when the patient who is liable to be detained is discharged from hospital. Patients who are on SCT are also entitled to be assessed for community services under this section	The RC can grant indefinite leave or more frequently leave for a specified length of time, which must be more than seven days. The RC must have considered the merits of a Community Treatment Order before using this section	The RC can order the willing discharge of an eligible patient who will be subject to recall if the patient does not comply with their treatment (ss.17 and 17E). Before an order can be made the AMHP must agree and do so in writing. The order can be renewed (s.20A). The initial period will be for six months with renewal at six months and thereafter annually	Either the nearest relative or the AMHP can apply plus two medical recommendations. If an AMHP makes the application the NR can object although if thought unreasonable this objection can be overruled by a County Court.
Notes	Section 117 services are provided under the remit of s.46 of the NHS and CCA 1990 and this requires that the LSSA carry out a two-stage assessment of needs for services. Once assessed as needing services the LSSA cannot charge for these services	This was designed to reduce the numbers of patients who were considered to be revolving-door patients. It allows the patient to leave hospital while still being subject to the powers of the Act. Non-compliant patients can be recalled and once back at hospital can be made subject to a CTO. Recalling automatically revokes the leave	This replaces supervised discharge under s.25A-25J, which was seldom used. These came into force after a series of cases that were high profile and showed that community care was not working. The new community treatment orders are referred to in the MHA 2007 as supervised community treatment. The patient can be recalled for up to 72 hours without affecting the order. Longer than this and the patient reverts to a detained patient status	Although this order can be used for Part 2 and Part 3 patients, mostly it is used in civil circumstances. The numbers of guardianship orders may increase as the new law broadens the power and extends the range of people to whom it might apply

decides if guardianship is suitable and will take into account all the circumstances of the case. Importance will be placed on reports made to the courts and the LSSA will be able to let the court know if it is prepared to receive the order and how it can exercise its responsibilities to the offender. The medical evidence is the same as for a civil order.

Care Programme Approach (CPA)

At present all mental health service users are entitled to the Care Programme Approach, which has two levels. However, in practice this has meant that mostly only those entitled to an enhanced level of CPA actually received a service. From 1 October 2008 the CPA will only apply to those at this level but will include all patients who are currently or have been recently detained under the MHA. This is called a 'refocused' CPA and the National Director for Mental Health in the forward of *Refocusing the CPA* stated the rationale as:

> the Care Programme Approach (CPA) is at the centre of a personalisation pro-
> cess, supporting individuals with severe mental illness to ensure their needs and
> choices remain central in what are often complex systems of care.

(DoH, 2008)

Service users eligible for CPA can expect:

- support from a trained CPA co-ordinator;
- a comprehensive multi-agency and multi-disciplinary assessment covering the full range of needs and risks;
- an assessment of their financial needs including direct payments;
- a comprehensive written care plan including risk assessments and contingency measures;
- the need for advocacy services assessed;
- at review consideration for ongoing CPA support;
- carers informed of their rights to their own assessment.

One of the consequences of the increasing complexity of systems of care and treatment is that they can become disjointed. Consequently a new shared computerised record system between primary and secondary care came into practice in 2010.

BEST PRACTICE

Applying for a warrant to search and remove patients section 135

This section looks at the process of obtaining a warrant from a Justice of the Peace (Magistrate) that enables the AMHP to be accompanied by a police constable to enter, by force if necessary, any premises specified in the warrant in which the person is believed to be, and thought fit, to remove that person to a place of safety that would then enable an application to be made under Part 2 of the MHA.

The AMHP applies for a warrant if they believe that the person is suffering from mental disorder and needs to convince the JP that there is a very real risk that the patient would resist the assessment and that the AMHP would encounter more risks that they would normally encounter in fulfilling their role. The AMHP may make the application either to a magistrate's court or to the magistrate in person if out of hours.

(Continued)

(Continued)

Best practice suggests that the AMHP needs to provide clearly documented evidence about why such a warrant is needed and a summary of the steps that they have taken prior to this application to undertake a mental health assessment with the identified person. In order to convince the JP, who will judge the application on its merits only, the AMHP needs to provide compelling reasons about why if the warrant is not granted there is a real risk that the person may hide themselves in the building, try to damage themselves or worse.

This needs the AMHP to consider the balance between responding to the perceived danger and the possible infringement of human rights obligation Article 8 the right to a private life. To help with this the AMHP should document the extent that police involvement will be needed and if this is proportionate to risks that are envisaged.

There is always the alternative that the police can attend the property with the AMHP and try to convince the patient to let them enter. If consent is withdrawn then legally they must leave the property. This means that the AMHP should figure out beforehand what the risks might be and make an application before entry is sought. The advantage is of course that the police constable can then use reasonable force to enter the premises.

The AMHP will know that even if the warrant is granted it does not have to be executed. So if when attending the property access is gained, even if rather surprisingly, the warrant need not be used but held as a form of insurance should the situation deteriorate.

These are situations where the good judgement of the AMHP comes into play, as each situation needs to be judged on its own merits and the strength of any relationship that the AMHP has with the local police. Often magistrates will hold meetings with local AMHPs to help to keep each other up to date.

S.136 mentally disordered persons found in public places

Tucked away under Part 10 is the above power that enables a constable to remove a person from a public place to a place of safety should the constable determine that the person is mentally ill and in need of immediate care or control (s.136 (1)). For a very readable and full account of one service user's experience through a mental health crisis to recovery you should read Gregory and Thompson's account (*Journal of Social Work Practice*, 2013).

In order for this section to be applied lawfully the following conditions need to be met:

- the person is found in a place to which the public have access;

- they appear to be suffering from a mental disorder;

- they are in need of immediate care or control; and

- it is in the interests of the person or to protect others that they are removed to a place of safety.

The first discussion point is what counts as a 'place to which the public have access', bearing in mind that the MHA goes no further than this rather general phrase. There is some evidence that the police who are often at the scene before anyone else use a degree of 'flexibility' with their interpretation of public place and it is not unknown for the officers to remove people from just outside their home, their garden or in some case from within their home. This is of course illegal as the law states that they must be found in a place to which the public has access.

What is quite surprising is the extent that police officers, usually with little or no mental health training, are quite good at recognising mental disorder when they see it (Lamb, 2002). Should the person satisfy the conditions above then they should be removed to a place of safety, which is defined by s.135 (6). It is also worth noting that technically the detention by the police is in fact an 'arrest' under the Police and Criminal Evidence Act. A problem arises when this detention or arrest can show on Criminal Record checks. This is one aspect the CQC are discussing with politicians with a view to amending this and avoiding employment difficulties for people who have been detained under this section. A place of safety is defined as:

> Residential accommodation provided by a local social services authority under Part 3 of the national Assistance Act 1948, a hospital as defined by the this Act, a police station, an independent hospital or care home for mentally disordered persons or any other suitable place the occupier of which is willing to receive the patient

(s.135 (6))

Well this seems to include pretty much everywhere including a domestic dwelling if the occupier is willing to receive the patient. It is to the Code of Practice that we must turn to seek enlightenment and note that it says that a police station should only be used on an exceptional basis and only if the patient presents 'an unmanageable high risk to others...' (E Para 10.21). Straightaway you are probably guessing that this is going to be a problem and if so you are right. This summer (2013) a senior police officer has hit out at this and correctly stated that police cells are not suitable for the majority of patients who need care and attention. There are no mental health services at the majority of police stations and detainees will have to wait, often for a considerable period of time, for services to attend. It was estimated that 11,000 patients were conveyed to a police station as a 'Place of Safety' most years (Gregory citing Bather et al., 2008). Not only are services not readily available but holding in a police cell potentially has a criminalising effect on service users.

Patients concerned in criminal proceedings or under sentence

The provisions in Part 3 of the Act enable the courts to order that offenders be detained in hospital for treatment, rather than prison.

Hospital orders (s. 37 and s. 41)

A small number of people may be admitted to hospital from the Crown Court. This may be pursuant to a Hospital Order made under section 37 of the MHA (for example), following their conviction for a criminal offence, or it may be as a result of their pleading that their mental state makes it impossible for them to have a fair trial. In the latter case, the patient will be subject to a Hospital Order by virtue of the Criminal Procedure (Insanity and Unfitness to Plead) Act 1991.

Where the court has convicted a person they can be remanded for psychiatric reports for up to 12 weeks before sentencing. Where mental disorder is apparent at the time of sentencing they may be admitted to a hospital under section 37, which is similar in extent to section 3 except that the applicant is in effect the Courts. If when making a Hospital Order, the Court decides that the public needs protection from serious harm it may also make a Restriction Order under section 41. The effect of a Restriction Order is that in most cases, the patient may not be discharged from hospital, transferred to another hospital or granted leave without the permission of the Secretary of State.

The concept of social vulnerability comes into play when a crime involves an older person who has limited capacity perhaps caused by mental illness or dementia. There is now a range of new offences under s.44 Mental Capacity Act 2005 (ill treatment or wilful neglect of a person who lacks capacity) and s.4 Fraud Act 2006 (this is called fraud by abuse of position).

Table 3.5 Detentions under Part 3 of the MHA (Source: HSCIC)

	2009–10	2010–11	2011–12	2012–13
NHS hospital	1431	1421	1444	1219
Independent hospital	760	717	686	569
ALL	2191	2138	2130	1788

The numbers of patients detained under Part 3 have decreased by 16% from 2011–12 to 2012–13, the only significant change over this period. Part 3 admissions represent about 6% of the overall admissions.

Treatment in hospital or the community

Medical treatment means a range of interventions including drug treatments, nursing care and therapeutic interventions, and could include behaviour modification and task-centred work. Where medical treatment is given, it should only be for the mental disorder that the patient is suffering. This provides a degree of safeguard for the patient but is open to interpretation and professional discretion. When a patient's life is under threat, the situation is far more complex. For example, the treatment of patients who have chronic eating disorders may necessitate 'forced' feeding, which is a physical treatment for a condition widely considered to have a psychological component. Where to draw the line between physical and mental disorder is usually a matter for professional decision-making and rulings through the courts. It is assumed that every adult patient has capacity to consent unless they lack capacity to make the decision, as defined in the MCA 2005.

Drug treatment

Patients who are detained under the MHA 1983 are subject to the provisions of Part 4 of the Act, which covers treatments that require consent and a second opinion (s.57), which is usually psycho-surgery; treatment that requires consent or a second opinion (s.58), usually medicine for a patient's mental disorder; and urgent treatment (s.62), which justifies departure from the requirements of s.58. The implications for practice are to be found in the Code of Practice. Medicine can be given to patients who are detained for treatment under s.3 or a hospital order (s.37) without their consent or a second opinion, for up to three months. This is known as the 'three month rule'. After three months, such treatment can only be given if its use has been approved by a second opinion appointed doctor (SOAD).

The medical treatment of informal patients in psychiatric hospitals in many ways mirrors that of patients in general hospitals and if they have the requisite capacity, such patients have the right to refuse treatment as well as discharge themselves without conditions (subject to s.5 holding powers). As the vast majority of capable patients are informal, the common law applies to their treatment for mental disorder in the same way as any other health problem. This means that every patient has the individual right to refuse treatment even if that refusal may be injurious to his or her health. However, the situation for patients who are subject to the detention powers in the MHA 1983 is different as they may in certain conditions be made to have treatment even though they object strongly to this form of intervention. The authority for this can be found in Part 4 of the MHA 1983, which applies only to detained patients. The policy of overriding the patient's wishes is justified when it is in either or both the patient's best interest or for the good of others. Although the use of such measures is provided with safeguards such as a second opinion, it is nevertheless seen by some as an example of the social-control function of psychiatry.

Elsewhere the range of medical interventions is discussed (Chapter 2). It is worth reflecting that prescribed drugs for the treatment of mental disorder account for around 25 % of all prescriptions issued through the NHS (Bartlett and Sandland, 2003, p.326). The treatment of a chronic disorder like schizophrenia is estimated to be over £1 billion pounds alone. Even with this huge spend, patients report varying degrees of satisfaction with these medications and relapse rate continues to be at a level that stretches service-level provision and the side effects cause some distress to many users.

For patients who are on SCT it is likely that their order will specify that they must continue to have treatment as directed by the RC and in particular to take prescribed medication.

Electro-convulsive treatment (ECT)

This treatment involves giving the patient electric shock treatment and is still in widespread use and usually considered when drug regimes appear not to work. It is an established method of treating people who have depression affective psychoses. ECT is always administered under anaesthetic and a muscle relaxant. Electrodes are placed on the temple and then a short electric shock is administered which produces a convulsion similar to an epileptic fit. Why this works for some patients and not for others remains a matter for speculation.

Many patients consent to this treatment but where patients do not and are detained they can, with certain safeguards, be given ECT against their wishes. Except in an emergency, a patient who is detained under the MHA but capable of consenting to ECT may only be given it with his consent. In the case of an incapable detained patient, ECT may only be given if it has been approved by a SOAD. If the patient is under 16 years of age and the situation is not considered urgent, SOAD approval will be required whether the patient is capable or incapable, and even if he isn't detained under the MHA. The length of treatment is usually 6 or 12 courses of treatment and approximately 20,000 patients have this treatment every year in the UK. Side effects can include memory impairment, often temporary, and confusion. Among older patients there are risks of strokes and heart attacks (Openmind, 1985). There is a possibility that the use of ECT against the wishes of detained patients contravenes the Human Rights Act but to date no legal action has been brought.

Psychosurgery

Although quite common at one time, with over 10,000 operations performed, this is now seldom carried out and when it is, it is subject to the investigation of a panel appointed by the Mental Health Act Commission and requires the patient's consent. Psychosurgery is irreversible.

Emergency treatment

This can mean the administration of medications and/or the restraint or seclusion of patients who are liable to be detained while in hospital. This is provided under s.62 and is limited to the minimum treatment necessary to respond to the emergency. This may not always be dramatic life-saving situations but could be for 'lesser emergencies'. Evidence suggests that from time to time this section has been used to include patients who are in hospital informally and presenting difficult behaviour on the hospital wards (Bartlett and Sandland, 2003).

Restraint may be necessary from time to time and should only be carried out by trained staff who are able to exercise minimal force that is consistent with resolution of the behaviour. The use of restraint is controversial and dates back to the use of straightjackets and other mechanical restraints. In the present time investigations and inquiries have thrown doubt upon the capabilities of some staff (MHAC, 2001).

When a patient's behaviour warrants it, he/she can be placed in seclusion, which involves the patient remaining in a room that is specially designated for the purpose and meets certain minimum requirements. While in this room the ward staff are required to not only observe the patient but also to record these observations and to arrange for medical review at periodic intervals. The MHAC reviews the use of seclusion and reports on this from time to time.

Part 9 offences

It is an offence for any person employed in a hospital or care home to ill-treat or wilfully neglect a patient who is receiving treatment as an inpatient or community patient (this includes guardianship). The penalty has recently been increased to a term not exceeding five years' imprisonment, which reflects the seriousness of this sort of offence and how it is viewed.

Part 10 Miscellaneous and supplementary

Under sections 135 and 136 of the Mental Health Act 1983 a police officer may remove a person who is believed or appears to be suffering from a mental disorder to a place of safety. Section 44 of the 2007 Act amends these sections of the 1983 Act to allow a person to be taken from one place of safety to one or more other places of safety during the 72-hour maximum overall period during which they may be detained under either of these two sections. This can be carried out by a police officer and AMHP, or someone authorised by either of them (Mental Health Act 2007 (Commencement No.5 and Transitional Provisions) Order 2008).

Getting out of hospital
Discharge

Informal patients cannot be subjected to compulsions of any kind and they may leave hospital when they wish (subject to the holding powers of s.5 of the MHA). In practice, patients should be advised to discuss discharge with their RC and others once they begin to feel better; this may be when medication has begun to work or when circumstances at home or in the community would allow them to leave hospital. This may necessitate social workers becoming involved in order to identify support services and systems that could be available for the patient and their families.

In some circumstances, a patient may be discharged from detention by his nearest relative (see s.23 of the MHA). It might, however, be possible for the RC to bar the patient's discharge, provided he does so in writing and within 72 hours of receipt of the nearest relative's order (s.25 (1) MHA).

A detained patient may apply for his discharge to the hospital managers and/or to the Mental Health Tribunal. A patient can seek discharge from both and being unsuccessful in one should not preclude success in the other. Tribunals are covered in more detail in Chapter 4.

Hospital managers' review

When a patient is detained under the MHA 1983 he/she can request that the hospital managers review the reasons for their continuing detention. Hospitals appoint a range of people who have had training and who have experience to act in this capacity. If the managers decide that the applicant is not suffering from a mental disorder or that he/she could live back in the community, they can order the discharge of the patient.

Regulation

The Health and Social Care Act 2008 established the Care Quality Commission (CQC) with the intention of providing an integrated approach to the regulation of the sector. In 2009 this 'super regulator' combined the functions of the former Healthcare Commission, Commission for Social Care Inspection and the Mental Health Act Commission. In Wales the duties of the MHAC have been taken over by the Health Inspectorate Wales.

This regulator will operate a 'light touch' for most providers but where significant failings are discovered will have the power to close wards or services. The important role of the Mental Health Act Commission in visiting patients detained under the Mental Health Act 1983 will be retained but it remains unclear whether it will continue to have the wider role it has forged in the protection of patients deprived of their liberty. The effectiveness of this 'super regulator' remains to be seen.

CHAPTER SUMMARY

This chapter has introduced you to the complex area of law and the inevitable responsibilities that are placed upon professionals. To deprive someone of their liberty is so serious that legal safeguards are essential. The role of the AMHP has been looked at in depth and through the case study you have covered one of the main processes through which people can be admitted to hospital, even if they object. Although some of the roles are specialised, it is essential that all social workers understand the basic provisions of the Mental Health Act and the corresponding Code of Practice. Remember that all law is experimental and subject to interpretation and change – it is your responsibility as a professional to keep up to date.

FURTHER READING

Fennell, P. (2007) *Mental Health: The new law*. Bristol: Jordan Publishing.

This is an excellent reference book. If you are interested in becoming an AMHP this is a key text for you study.

For the Mental Health Act 2007 itself, see:

Department of Health (2008) *Mental Health Act 1983 Draft Reference Guide to the Mental Health Act 1983 as amended by the Mental Health Act 2007*. Can be downloaded (beware: over 300 pages) *from* **www.dh.gov.uk/publications**

For a scholarly discussion of Community Treatment Orders set alongside the findings from a systematic review of existing studies on Community Treatment Orders, a report well worth reading is the report by

King's College London, Institute of Psychiatry (2007), *International Experiences of using Community Treatment Orders*, which can be obtained either on the web or from the Section of Evidence-based Mental Health, Health Services Research Department, PO Box 32, Institute of Psychiatry, King's College London, De Crespigny Park, London SE5 8AF. Their web address is: **www.iop.kcl.ac.uk/news/**

For the latest report on the evaluation of Community Treatment Orders see

Burns, T., Rugkåsa, J., Molodynski, A., Dawson, J., Yeeles, K., Vazquez-Montes, M., Voysey, M., Sinclair, J. and Priebe, S (2013). Community treatment orders for patients with psychosis (OCTET): a randomised controlled trial. *Lancet* (2013; in press). See more at: **www.thementalelf.net/mental-health-conditions/schizophrenia/community-treatment-orders-fail-to-reduce-psychiatric-readmissions-for-people-with-psychosis/#sthash.84Pq0JWf.dpuf**

For the hungry statistician, your first port of call should be the **Information Centre for Social Care.** They provide an annual publication, which summarises information about people detained under the 1983 Mental Health Act in NHS facilities, including high-security psychiatric hospitals, and independent hospitals. It includes figures for the period 1996–97 to 2006–07. Their web address is **www.ic.nhs. Uk/statistics-and-data-collections/mental-health/mental-health-act/in-patients**

For information and facts about numbers of detentions **www.hscic.gov.uk/article/3668/Mental-Health-Act-detentions-top-50000-a-year**

For a detailed and thorough understanding of mental capacity turn to **Brown, R., Barber, P. and Martin, D.** (2009) *The Mental Capacity Act 2005* (Second edition). Exeter: Learning Matters (Post-Qualifying Services)

For further information about social circumstances reports read **Curran, C., Golightley, M. and Fennell, P.** (2010) *Social Circumstances Reports for Mental Health Tribunals,* **Legal Action** Part 1 June and Part 2 July.

WEBSITES

Free downloads can be requested from the institutional repository at the University of Lincoln using **http://eprints.lincoln.ac.uk/4349/** for Part One and **http://eprints.lincoln.ac.uk/4350/** for Part Two.

Alternatively this can be accessed through a very useful web-site **www.hempsons.co.uk/news/hempsons-in-print/article/mental-health-tribunals-legal-action-journal/b2016582f5/?tx_ttnews[backPid]=579**

Chapter 4

The policy and legal context for practice Part 2: Mental Health Tribunals; Mental Capacity

A C H I E V I N G   A   S O C I A L   W O R K   D E G R E E

Knowledge of legal rules and their application to practice are features in the social work subject benchmark statements, which universities must meet. This chapter will help you to develop the following capabilities from the **Professional Capabilities Framework:**

- **Professionalism**
  Identify and behave as a professional social worker committed to professional development.

- **Rights, justice and economic wellbeing**
  Advance human rights and promote social justice and economic wellbeing.

- **Knowledge**
  Apply knowledge of social sciences, law and social work practice theory.

- **Intervention and skills**
  Use judgement and authority to intervene with individuals, families and communities to promote independence, provide support and prevent harm, neglect and abuse.

It will also introduce you to the following standards as set out in the 2008 social work subject benchmark statement:

4.3	Defining principles.
5.0	Subject knowledge and understanding and skills.
5.1.1	Social work services, service users and carers.
5.1.2	Service delivery context.
5.1.3	Values and ethics.
5.2	Subject-specific skills and other skills.
5.5.3	Analysis and synthesis.

Introduction

This chapter has two quite distinct parts to it. The first is about what you need to know about mental health tribunals, who does what and what your role could be at such tribunal hearings. The notorious Ian Brady, the 'moors murderer', is currently detained at a high secure unit and his appeal to the Tribunal was uniquely held in public, at his request, raising some fundamental issues that are dealt with in this part. The second part introduces the complex world of mental capacity – the law, codes of practice and case law have all intermingled to make a social worker's role in this area of work worthy of the discussion raised in the chapter.

Part 1: Mental Health Tribunal (s.65)

The First-tier Tribunal (Mental Health) hears applications and references for people detained under the Mental Health Act 1983 (as amended by the Mental Health Act 2007) and replaces the Mental Health Review Tribunal. The jurisdiction covers the whole of England. Wales has a separate provision. They represent a serious attempt to provide the patient and family with judicial review of whether detention is warranted. The Tribunal sits within the Health, Education and Social Care Chamber of the First-tier Tribunal.

Tribunals are independent judicial bodies that decide if a patient should continue to be detained or remain subject to a community treatment order or be discharged into the community. Previously known as a mental health review tribunal the name suggested, erroneously, that its role was to review the original decision to detain the patient when in reality it is about whether the patient should continue to be detained and what resources and facilities are available to support the patient should the decision be made to discharge. The outcome of the Panel should be a balanced judgement, often weighing up the rights of the individual against the best interests of the individual and the public. Mental health tribunals are not a venue for a case conference or an informal meeting. Attendees will usually be witnesses, and they need to be aware of protocol when attending hearings, and to act in a professional manner that shows respect to the hearing and to the service user.

The hospital managers (NHS trust or independent hospital registered to take detained patients) or if subject to guardianship, the local social services authority (LSSA), must justify the need for the continued use of the Act. The Act sets out the circumstances in which an MHT can discharge a detained patient. When granting a patient his discharge, the MHT has the power to defer the date on which it will take effect. Alternatively, and with a view to facilitating a patient's discharge in the future, the MHT may recommend that he be given leave of absence, transferred to another hospital or into guardianship, or be made subject to SCT. Each MHT has three members: a legal member who is its president, a medical member who is usually a consultant psychiatrist, and a lay member. The Ministry of Justice appoints all members. These are remunerated positions and reflect the seriousness that is rightly given to the work of the tribunal. Each member must consider the case on its individual merits.

Social workers should always remind the patient that they are entitled to be represented by a solicitor with specialist mental health experience, absolutely free of charge under the legal aid scheme. This is especially important as the patient/NR may be worried about paying the fee. The solicitor may decide to involve an expert witness, e.g. independent psychiatrist, social worker or psychologist. In the case of long-term patients detained under s.3 who do not apply to the tribunal within the first six months, the hospital manager must refer the case to the tribunal.

In all cases a Social Circumstances Report (SCR) will be required and a social worker or a community psychiatric nurse (CPN) or therapist who need not be an AMHP can compile these. Over recent years there has been some concern about the quality and information contained in some social circumstances reports. These concerns are generally about the often out-of-date information and the inclusion of material that is irrelevant to the needs of the tribunal. Members report that plans for the patient post discharge are seldom as full as the members would like and consequently may not assist the tribunal.

Rules and directions govern the contents of these reports. The Mental Health Review Tribunal Rules 1983, which formerly applied in England and Wales, have now been replaced by discrete Tribunal Rules for each country. In England, the provision of information in mental health cases is governed by the Tribunal Procedure (First-tier Tribunal) (Health, Education and Social Care Chamber) Rules 2008, and by the Practice Direction, which was issued in 2008, and revised in 2013.

Purpose of a SCR

The main purpose of a SCR is to provide the tribunal with 'hard' evidence of the patient's circumstances if discharged from hospital, in particular, what medical, social services and other support will be available in the community, together with 'soft' – but also potentially significant – evidence about the views of the nearest relative and non-professional others who play a significant part in the patient's care, the patient's own views and an assessment of the patient's strengths and positive factors. The SCR should provide evidence of planned aftercare, in line with the guidance in the MHA Codes of Practice for England and Wales on the duty to provide aftercare under MHA 1983 s.117 and the English and Welsh policy guidance on the Care Programme Approach (CPA).

SCRs and human rights

Article 5(4) of the European Convention requires speedy access to independent review of the lawfulness of detention before a court or tribunal with the power to order discharge. In England, the task of reviewing the lawfulness of detention is exercised by the mental health tribunal (and in Wales by the Mental Health Review Tribunal). The Tribunal panel needs to determine the 'Winterwerp criteria' that there is objective medical evidence that the patient continues to suffer from mental disorder and that this is sufficient to justify continuing detention and is a proportionate response to the patient's situation. This includes looking at aftercare arrangements for a patient if they were discharged and the extent that these could support the patient to the extent that care can be provided outside of the hospital.

The 2013 Practice Direction

The provision of a social circumstances report (SCR) for a mental health tribunal has been a legal requirement since the Mental Health Act 1959. Since 2008 there have been separate mental health tribunals for England and Wales. In England, the provision of information in mental health cases by the responsible authority (RA) and the Secretary of State for Justice is governed by the ***Tribunal Procedure (First-tier Tribunal) (Health, Education and Social Care Chamber) Rules 2008 (the Tribunal Procedure Rules) SI No 2699*** Rule 32(5) and **a new Practice Direction** which is effective from 28 October 2013 (the 2013 PD) that replaces earlier versions. SCR writers must provide appropriate reports, depending on the type of tribunal case. The 2013 PD sets out what information and reports are required for the following cases; **Part A:** In-patients; **Part B:** Community patients – community treatment order (CTO); **Part C:** Guardianship patients; **Part D:** Conditionally discharged patients; and **Part E:** Patients below 18 years (Child and Adolescent Mental Health Services – CAMHS patients).

The completion of these reports is a statutory requirement and they provide the tribunal with information about the patient and their social circumstances and sits alongside the responsible clinician's report and an in-patient report. If you are writing a report the first step should be a careful reading of the 2013 PD. Should for whatever reason the SCR is not provided or the information is insufficient this could result in a delay in discharging the patient with possible distress for the patient and others.

SCRs: content and layout

The quality of the SCR (Curran, et al., 2014) is crucial as it reflects on the importance that the compiler has placed on the service user and the judicial process. The list of headings is lengthy and the information needs to be as good as it possibly can be. All reports should be paginated and prepared specifically for the tribunal. Although it has to be a matter of personal preference as to whether the SCR goes further than meeting the statutory requirements in the latest Practice Direction it is suggested that this may not meet the needs of the tribunal and writers should consider the importance of this report and the following suggestions. The headings are set out below with (RR) identifying the regulatory requirement and the remainder suggestions.

- (RR) SCR It is a regulatory requirement that: *The statement provided to the tribunal must **include** an up-to-date social circumstances report **prepared for the tribunal**.* If several weeks have elapsed since the first SCR, the report writer should submit an addendum, thus ensuring it is up to date on the day of the hearing. If the SCR relates to a restricted patient (for example, MHA 1983 ss.37 and 41) the addendum report should be submitted several days before the hearing so that the Secretary of State (i.e. via the Mental Health Unit at the Ministry of Justice) may comment.
- Patient's full name: Is s/he known by any other names?
- Date of birth/age.
- Ward: Community address if under a community treatment order (CTO).
- Status: For example, married, single, divorced.
- MHA status: For example, ss.3, 34, 41.

- Date of original detention.

- Referral or an application date: Indicate if this is a referral or an application to the tribunal.

- Address at time of admission: i.e., home address if known.

- SCR writer: Include the full name and title, for example, care coordinator,

- Approved mental health professional, community psychiatric nurse, social worker, occupational therapist and place of work (for example, assertive outreach team or community mental health team). Will the SCR writer remain involved with the patient after the hearing date?

- Professional relationship to patient: For example, care coordinator and length of involvement.

- Responsible clinician: Name and length of time treating the patient.

- Care coordinator: Full name, title, contact details and date of most recent contact.

- Responsible authority/primary care trust: For example, highlight commissioning authority or regional secure commissioning team involvement.

- Index offence: If appropriate and whether Multi-Agency Public Protection Arrangements (MAPPA) involved, the sex offenders register, etc.

- Sources of information: That forms the basis of the SCR, for example, under the refocused Care Programme Approach (CPA) and other meetings, patient's electronic/case records, with relevant dates.

- Chronology: Provision of previous admission dates in a chronological table is very helpful. Indicate the date the present authority to detain was renewed, periods of MHA 1983 s17 leave or a detailed CTO history.

- Current admission: For example, the writer's understanding of events leading to admission, how the patient has responded to the detention and other significant events, for example, s.17 leave.

- Brief psychiatric history: Include the patient's past MHA history (a chronological table is recommended). The success or failure of any previous discharge arrangements should be described – what lessons were learnt?

- (RR) Home and family circumstances: This information enables the tribunal to gauge the level of family support or otherwise.

- (RR) Nearest relative (where the patient is unrestricted): Summarise the nearest relative's views. In order to identify the correct nearest relative, it is useful to list close family members (i.e., spouse/partner, children, parents: MHA 1983 s.26) and specify dates of birth/age and relationship to the patient. A chronological family table is strongly recommended.

- (RR) Views of any person with a substantial part in the care of the patient.

- Independent mental health advocate: Include any details relating to advocacy input.

- (RR) Patient's views: Include the patient's concerns, hopes and beliefs in relation to the tribunal proceedings.

- (RR) Employment opportunities: The patient's education and employment history should be included. Employment is an important part of daily living and effective after-care planning should address this issue and also consider available leisure options.

- (RR) Housing facilities available: i.e., what housing facilities are actually available if the tribunal discharges the patient, for example, location, type of tenancy, etc.

Quality of SCRs

Anselm Eldergill in *Mental Health Review Tribunals: Law and practice* (1997) states that the most common fault with SCRs is simply that the writer was obviously unaware of the required content of such reports. Where SCRs fail to comply with the relevant Practice Direction, presently December 2013, i.e., providing insufficient information to reach an informed decision, the tribunal may be compelled to adjourn the case (with all that that involves in terms of resources, impact on the patient, his/her family and legal representatives, health care professionals and the tribunal) and 'direct' the responsible authority to furnish a supplementary SCR (Tribunal Procedure Rules r5(3)(d)).

The most recent report from the Care Quality Commission (CQC) (2011) related to 'Patients' experiences of the First-tier Tribunal (Mental Health)', many respondents

> *...expressed concern about the provision of information ... and.... many complained about limited access to reports, which form an important part of the evidence on which the tribunal bases its decision. Nearly a third believed they had not seen any of these reports ... [and]... a few commented ... they received the reports too late to put together a proper response....*

The report (p.23) recommends that professionals providing reports to the tribunal should ensure reports are provided in good time before the hearing, in compliance with the Tribunal Rules and practice direction.

Non-disclosure of information

There may be occasions when you feel there is specific information they wish to draw to the attention of the Tribunal, but don't want the patient to know. The Tribunal decision as to whether or not to grant such a request for non-disclosure is governed by Rule 14(2)(a). The bar to grant such a request is high, and the Tribunal must be ' ... satisfied that such disclosure would be likely to cause that person or some other person serious harm; and ... having regard to the interest of justice, that it is proportionate to give such a direction'. If the tribunal is asked to consider non-disclosure on this basis, care must be taken to 'provide that evidence to the tribunal in a separate document, clearly marked to that effect'. Such a request should be submitted (except for s.2 cases), in advance of the hearing to the Tribunal administration centre.

Attendance at tribunals

Mental Health Act Code of Practice, para 32.30 states, '... It is important that other people who prepare reports submitted by the responsible authority attend the hearing to provide further up-to-date information about the patient, including (where relevant) their home circumstances and the aftercare available in the event of a decision to discharge the patient'. This is important because the report may raise issues on which the Tribunal will need to question the author in order to obtain sufficient information to make its decision. Also, by the time of the hearing there may have been further developments, including improvement in the patient's condition or appropriate housing facilities becoming available, which may not have been apparent when the report was written. For the patient to have a fair hearing it is important that this up-to-date information is available in order to avoid unnecessary adjournments.

(Adapted from Curran, Golightley and Fennel, 2014)

Tribunals become a national obsession!

Hard to believe but in the summer of 2013 Tribunals suddenly went public, well one particular one did. I was lucky enough to be in attendance during some of the hearing which offered the rare chance to see a political dance acted out and to reflect on the nature and extent of the hearing. The Mental Health Tribunal was held under the Tribunal procedure (First-tier Tribunal) Health Education & Social Care Chamber Rules 2008.

The notorious moors murderer Ian Brady launched a legal fight to be allowed to starve himself to death. In order to advance his wishes he had to get the Tribunal to accept that he was no longer mentally ill and therefore should be discharged. He argued that 50 years held 'in captivity' was long enough and wanted to return to prison where he thought he would enjoy greater freedoms and privileges.

His appearance at the mental health tribunal – via video link – is the first time he has been seen in public for decades. The Tribunal was originally set for July 2012 but after Brady developed a medical condition it was postponed until summer 2013. The arrangements were that the hearing would be heard in Ashworth and relayed to the Civil Justice Centre Manchester for members of the public to watch the proceedings. No member of the public was allowed to the hearing room at Ashworth. I was one of the members of the public who sat rather transfixed during some of the hearing alongside relatives of one of Brady's victims.

The issue revolved around the issue of whether or not Brady could be judged mentally ill within the meaning of the Mental Health Act. An eight-day hearing, in which Brady gave evidence on the last day, was thought necessary in order to determine his status. If successful, the 75 year old hoped that he could be moved to a Scottish jail and be allowed to starve to death.

Currently he is detained at Ashworth maximum security hospital in Merseyside. He has been there since 1985, when he was sectioned under the Mental Health Act. He is believed to be the longest-serving compulsory admission patient to be held in a secure facility.

The relatives of his victims have repeatedly said they wish him to be kept alive.

Brady, whose accomplice Myra Hindley died in 2002, has been on hunger strike for 13 years. For all of that time he has been fed by nasal feeding tube. Although evidence given at the Tribunal and dismissed as irrelevant by Brady suggests that he also supplements this regime with daily toast and 'cup-a-soup' snacks.

Although sensationalised, the issues this tribunal raises are fundamental and of relevance to all of us in the mental health field. Who defines who is mentally ill? Should a convicted murderer be allowed to terminate his own life?

In a Kafkaesque experience lawyers for both sides argued about the nature of mental illness and treatment and finally agreed that Brady suffered from a narcissistic personality disorder. Where they did disagree was if he also had paranoid schizophrenia. You can guess which side argued which.

Are people mad or bad? Brady when giving evidence claimed that the murders were 'recreational' and an 'existential experience' but was this evidence of badness or madness?

Can you feign mental illness? After all the Rosehan study seemed to suggest that this was entirely possible (1973). Brady claimed that by using the Stanislavski method acting techniques he was able dupe some of the country's eminent psychiatrists. But having once thought that life would be better in a hospital, albeit a high secure one like Ashworth, he realised the error that he made and now wants to go back to prison about which he was increasingly lyrical during the tribunal. He talked about the relationships that he had with some notorious criminals like the 'great train robbers' and their likes.

After being 'cared' for at Ashworth Brady has admitted that he doesn't expect to be released, which for him is realistic, but he wants to be free to choose when to end his life. As a detained patient he is being force fed under the legal framework of the MHA. Is this appropriate?

The actual costs of his care over the last period in Ashworth are estimated to be about £14 million. Too much or value for money? Alan Bennett, the brother of one of Brady's victims, was present every day at the Tribunal and was quoted in the *Guardian* as 'I am happiest knowing that Brady will be at his unhappiest. I know he hates Ashworth and I cannot be sure he would feel the same about any other place he may be sent to.'

After four days of the hearing and several weeks after the decision was delivered.

> *The Tribunal has concluded that Mr. Ian Stewart Brady continues to suffer from a mental disorder which is of nature and degree which makes it appropriate for him to continue to receive medial treatment and that is is necessary for his health and safety and for the protection of other persons that he should receive such treatment in hospital and that appropriate medical treatment is available for him.*

Judge Robert Ashton, Tribunal president, 28 June 2013
(Mental Health Law Online)

This case study can be useful in helping to understand the dynamic between understanding and intervention. One of the arguments used by counsel in the Brady Tribunal went along the lines that he was refusing to co-operate with the psychiatric team at Ashworth, which they interpreted as evidence of continuing mental illness (in this case paranoid schizophrenia), and that if you are hearing voices or indeed hallucinating then this must be a sign of your illness rather simply a personal characteristic. If you follow this through then you come to the irreducible truth that illness can only be defined by a medically qualified person and as such only treated by a similarly qualified person.

In Brady's case three experts testified that although he does have a personality disorder of the narcissistic type he did not have paranoid schizophrenia.

Regulation

Who monitors the operation of the Mental Health Act has fallen to a relatively new body that has already come under close scrutiny and there are lingering doubts about the likelihood of this body being able to live up to our expectations.

The Health and Social Care Act 2008 established the Care Quality Commission (CQC) with the intention of providing an integrated approach to the regulation of the sector. In 2009 this 'super regulator' combined the functions of the former Healthcare Commission, Commission for Social Care Inspection and the Mental Health Act Commission. In Wales the duties of the MHAC have been taken over by the Health Inspectorate Wales.

This regulator operates a 'light touch' for most providers but where significant failings are discovered they have the power to close wards or services. The important role of the Mental Health Act Commission in visiting patients detained under the Mental Health Act 1983 was retained but it remains unclear whether it will continue to have the wider role it has forged in the protection of patients deprived of their liberty. Make sure that you read the annual report of the CQC available as a free download or by request as a hard copy for while it might sound like a rather dull document it is anything but and contains some very useful information.

For further reading and recommended websites, see page 115 at the end of this chapter.

Part 2: Introduction to Mental Capacity Act and Deprivation of Liberty Safeguards

This Part introduces you to the complexities of mental capacity or lack of it and the protection provided by the relevant legislation and procedures. The aim is to enable you to understand the key components of the legislation and the Code of Practice and to grasp how people come within their provisions.

Why was a law on capacity needed?

The Mental Capacity Act (MCA) 2005 has consolidated human rights law for people who may lack capacity to make their own decisions and it is designed to promote the empowerment of individuals and to protect their rights. The law is founded on five basic principles that guide decision-making for the estimated 2 million people who may lack capacity in some aspect of their lives (SCIE, October 2013. p.1).

Many social workers and other professionals will from time to time be concerned about their liability under law if they intervene and make decisions for some people that subsequently turns out to have a negative effect. However, under the MCA if the social worker meets the legal requirements then it is taken for granted that the decision made by the social worker will be as if the person concerned had made the decision himself or herself. For large numbers of people their capacity to make certain decisions about their life is affected either on a temporary or on a permanent basis. The Mental Capacity Act covers situations where someone is unable to make a decision because the way their mind or brain works is affected, for instance, by illness or disability, or the effects of drugs or alcohol. A lack of mental capacity could be due to:

- a mental health problem;

- brain injury or stroke damage;

- confusion, drowsiness or unconsciousness because of an illness or the consequences of treatment for it;

- dementia;

- learning disability;

- substance misuse.

The MCA applies to everyone who works in England and Wales in the health and social care sector and is supporting the care, treatment and support of people who are over 16 years old and may lack the capacity to make their own decisions. Note that some parts such as the Deprivation of Liberty Safeguards only apply to people who are 18 years and older. The thinking behind this legislation was to introduce a single and coherent framework that would put the service user at the heart of the decision-making process and introduce some important safeguards for them.

Key principles of the MCA

The MCA has five key principles that help to understand the fundamental nature of the Act and just what values underpin the legislation. These are found in Part 1 of the MCA and can summarised as follows:

- Every adult has the right to make their own decisions unless it is determined that they lack the mental capacity at that time to do so. This is regardless of age, disability, etc.

- Sometimes with support and assistance people can be enabled to make their own decisions and every effort should be made to try this out and even if a lack of capacity is established to involve the person as much as possible. Are there different times of day when it is easier for a person to understand about a decision? Can they be helped with visual representation of the issue?

- Respect for other people's values and beliefs should be upheld and this includes the right to make eccentric or strange decisions including ones that you might not make for yourself.

- Anything that is done on behalf of a person who lacks capacity must be shown to be in their 'best interests'.

- Before the act is done, or the decision made, it must be considered if the purpose for which it is needed can be as effectively achieved in way that is less restrictive of the person's rights and freedom of action (Part 1, 1.6 the MCA 2005). Thus the principle of the least restrictive option applies with the qualifier that it is about effectiveness of the action.

What is capacity?

Mental capacity is the ability to make a decision which can affect everyday decisions, like when to get up, what to wear and when it is necessary to go to the doctors. It also refers to making decisions that could have legal consequences either for them-selves or others like making a will or agreeing to have medical treatment. Capacity is assessed on a single issue and on the balance of probabilities and the safeguards that have been introduced are often referred to as bridging the ***Bournewood gap.***

Section 2 of the MCA 2005 states that a person lacks capacity if they are unable to make a decision, and sets out the following as a test. Is the person able to do the following?

- Understand the information that is needed to be able to make a decision.

- Retain the information.

- Use that information when trying to decide what to do.

- Communicate the decision whether by talking, using sign language or other means (called the 'statutory test').

Every effort should be made to assist the person to communicate before deciding that they lack capacity on the grounds that they have poor communication. The guidance suggests that very few people lack capacity on this ground only. Those in a coma might of course be such people. If faced with this situation seek specialist input and always record in your notes how you came to the conclusion that the person lacked capacity to make this specific decision.

Once a decision is made it can of course be challenged either by the person who you have assessed or by their representative. There is a specific Code of Practice for the MCA (2007) which provides guidance to all those who make decisions on behalf of adults who lack capacity. This is helpful in identifying the various channels that can be used to resolve disputes. If this fails the person or their representative may seek a rul-ing from the Court of Protection.

Anybody who claims that an individual lacks capacity should be able to provide proof. They need to be able to show, on the balance of probabilities, that the individual lacks capacity to make a particular decision, at the time it needs to be made (section 2(4)). This means being able to show that it is more likely than not that the person lacks capacity to make the decision in question.

(4.10 Code of Practice, MCA ,2007)

Excluded decisions

While the MCA covers a wide range of decisions or actions that can be taken on behalf of people who lack capacity to make the decision themselves there are important exclusions to the scope of this section of the Act. Decisions that are not covered by the MCA include marriage or civil partnership, divorce, sexual relationships, adoption and voting, either because they are so personal or because they are already covered by other legislation. More information can be found on pages 16–17 of the relevant Code of Practice.

When considering if a decision is included or excluded you need to take into account the capacity of the person and even if from the outset you are clear that the decision is excluded an assessment of the person's capacity should be made. If after this the person remains vulnerable then this could be used as a justification of action made in order to protect a vulnerable person from abuse or exploitation.

Limitations of the MCA

The person preserves voting rights and there is no scope for anyone to vote on their behalf even if they are sure of the way that the person would vote if they were capable of so doing.

Similarly nothing in the Act provides for the unlawful killing whether by assisted suicide or other means of a person who has limited capacity.

Legal protection from liability for health and social care workers

The MCA offers limited protection for health and social care workers providing that you have observed the principles of the Act and that you have carried out an assessment of capacity and reasonably believe that you have acted in the best interests of the person. This is important as it does provide you with protection when carrying out actions that the person may not consent to. These include, but are not limited to, personal care including dressing and hygiene, eating and drinking and helping people to walk, changes in residence. Naturally you should make clear records of the steps that you have taken and the reasons behind why you did so even thought the person was objecting.

The issue of restraint

This is an area, which at first glance, you may feel uncomfortable about as it runs contrary to fundamental values that underpin social work yet there may be occasions when this is the best option open to you or to carers. Restraint covers a wide range of actions from the use of 'cot sides' to stop someone getting out of bed or a restriction on where someone could go. In order to comply with the MCA you need to 'reasonably believe' that that the action is in the best interest of the person.

Statement of wishes, feelings, beliefs and values

These statements are used typically by someone who has a degenerative condition and wants people who will be going to care for him/her to take into account things that they feel strongly about. This might include vegetarian or kosher diet and they will record this and it needs to be placed onto their file. Now, unlike living wills, this does not have the force of the law behind it but you should take this into account when you decide what is in the best interests of the person concerned. If you decide that it is in the person's best interests to do other than they have requested you need to record this in the event of this decision being challenged.

Why does there need to be Deprivation of Liberty Safeguards?

The Deprivation of Liberty Safeguards provide a legal framework to prevent breaches of Article 5 of the European Convention of Human Rights (ECHR), which states that everyone has the right to liberty and security and that no one shall be deprived of his liberty except in accordance with a procedure prescribed by law covering the lawful detention of persons of unsound mind.

The safeguards were necessary to protect people who lack capacity and therefore are not capable at the moment of making a decision about their care and who need to be deprived of their liberty in order to protect them. The Mental Capacity Act 2005 Deprivation of Liberty Safeguards (MCA DOLS) came into practice on 1 April 2009 and provides a legal framework to prevent the unlawful detention of liberty that can be tested before law and that meets the necessary human rights legislation.

Prior to the introduction of this legislative change informal admission under the MHA 1983 s. 131 was used not just for those who agreed to admission but also for incapable patients who were not actively resisting or protesting against their admission. Such a course was felt to be lawful under the common-law doctrine of necessity.

However this assumption was challenged with *HL v United Kingdom*, when the European Court of Human Rights (ECtHR) noted that where a person is subject to such a degree of control over his basic human needs that he is deprived of his liberty, this will only be lawful if there is an adequate 'procedure prescribed by law'. The conclusion they reached was that in the case of incapable patients Informal Admission under s.131 was not such a procedure. HL was an autistic man who could not speak and it was clear that although he was held as an informal patient, if he decided to leave he would have been prevented from doing so. He was at the time admitted to a hospital run by the Bournewood Trust and the nature of his care was such that the ECHR found, deprived him of his liberty. This situation is unlawful because the common law of necessity is too vague and has too few effective safeguards to comply with Articles 5(1) and 5(4) of the ECHR. Thus HL was *de facto* detained and the DoLS represent the government's attempt to remedy the problem that the Bournewood case highlighted.

As a result the MCA applies to people who are admitted to a NHS hospital, an independent hospital or another residential facility who lack the capacity to consent to their admission but who are nonetheless, deprived of liberty (Fennell, 2007).

For any such deprivation of liberty to be lawful, it will have to have been authorised under the formal procedures set out in the DoLS. There are five points that you should understand.

- Always assume that someone has capacity.

- Understand what is meant by the capacity to make a decision at a particular time.

- Treat everyone equally irrespective of age, ethnicity or gender.

- Support the person to make their own decision whenever possible.

- Assess capacity using a two-stage test:

    ○ Does the person have an impairment of the mind or brain or is there some sort of disturbance affecting the way that their mind or brain works?

    ○ If so, does that impairment or disturbance mean that the person is unable to make the decision in question at the time that it needs to be made?

If in the case of a particular adult, no authorisation has been obtained under the DoLS, a deprivation of liberty will only be lawful if:

- it is the subject of an order made by the court of protection under s.16 (2) of the MCA; or

- an application has been made to the court and, in the meantime, it is necessary to save the person's life or prevent serious deterioration in his condition.

Deprivation of Liberty Safeguards

From the outset the term 'deprivation of liberty' might strike you as a rather negative term and perhaps you would support a recommendation to switch this to 'protective care' as proposed by the Mental Health Alliance (Mental Health Alliance briefing paper). However, deprivation of liberty is what we have and it is one of the three ways in which a person who lacks capacity can lawfully be deprived of their liberty and is the process most likely you will come across or are familiar with. There is a good argument that the principles are such that all social workers should be familiar with them as these will assist in their everyday social work practice.

However, although knowledge of DoLS is now fairly universal amongst healthcare providers, being alive to the need to apply them varies considerably. For example, those working in acute hospital settings are likely to encounter fewer DoLS referrals than, say, those working in the provision of long-term care. The result is that there is variation with the application of DoLS and the prospect of some patients slipping through the DoLS net.

The DoLS are covered in Schedule A1 'Hospital and care home residents: Deprivation of Liberty', which clearly describes the procedure for depriving a person of their liberty when they are in a care home or hospital. Where they are the managing authority they need to identify the person who is being, or likely to be deprived of their liberty within the next 28 days and apply for authorisation to do so using Schedule A1 Para 24. This request is made to the Supervisory Body. There is standard authorisation used when it is possible to operate the process over a period not exceeding 28 days and for urgent authorisations the time limit is up to 7 days.

Any application for an authorisation needs to be made in writing and ideally on the prescribed form. The information that is needed is to be found in the Regulations (2008) for the MCA. These are fairly obvious and include name and gender, age (must be believed to be over 18 years) and a range of information about medical assessment and treatments, existing care plans, existence of any advance directives, whether the person is subject to hospital, community or guardianship regime, etc.

Has an unauthorised deprivation of liberty occurred?

Para 69 of Schedule A1 permits requests to be made to the supervisory body to decide if an unauthorised deprivation of liberty is occurring. This at first glance may seem such an easy question to ask but in reality some of these decisions are on a knife-edge. There is often a tension between restraint and deprivation of liberty such that some cases have gone to the courts for decision. Consider, if you will, does a locked door constitute a deprivation of liberty? Well in a ruling the courts decided that the answer must be qualified by the extent that the person is able to move through the 'locked door' so we see the installation of key pad doors with the number printed alongside the door. The courts have judged that the difference between deprivation of and restriction are a matter of degree or intensity and not one of nature or substance (case law *Guzzardi v Italy* (1980) 3 EHRR 33).

What authority is responsible?

There are two legal entities that are important to understand:

Managing authorities who provide care and who need authorisation to provide care that amounts to detention. In the case of a private hospital or care home, it is the 'person registered' who is the managing authority, whereas for the NHS, it is the NHS body responsible for the management of the hospital.

Supervisory bodies were from 1 April 2013 transferred from the primary care trusts to local authorities under the provision made in the Health and Social Care Act (HSCA) 2012. This means that NHS and private hospitals now have to forward applications for authorisation to the local authority, which must organise assessment to determine, among other things, if detention is in the best interests of the patient and issue authorisations if appropriate. Each local authority will have a DoLS office and this office will need to work with hospitals to develop effective communication lines and to ensure accurate and up-to-date information is held in secure and safe manner.

The DoLS teams are establishing themselves as 'expert' in providing care and support to vulnerable people within a human rights approach.

Best interest assessors

If a person has been assessed as lacking in capacity then any action that is made on their behalf must be made in accordance with principle 4 and to be in their best interests. This will be familiar to you as it is essentially a codified form of common law. However you need to note that the determination of what counts as best interests is a mandatory process. The process to be used is set out on a checklist of common factors that need to be taken into consideration. The checklist is to be found in Chapter 5 of the Code of Practice.

The College of Social Work in March 2013 set out six capabilities that councils need to consider when appointing best interest assessors (BIAs) for people who fall under the DoLS. Best interest assessors are mostly social workers although they could be nurses, occupational therapists or psychologists with two years' post-qualifying experience and have completed an approved BIA course.

The College capabilities framework at present is not mandatory but is a set of good practice standards. It is up to the supervisory body to decide whether to adopt these capabilities but the informed view is that they will be adopted. A BIA should have the ability to:

1. apply in practice, and maintain knowledge of relevant legal and policy frameworks;

2. work in a manner congruent with the presumption of capacity;

3. take all practical steps to help someone make a decision;

4. balance a person's right to autonomy and self-determination with their right to safety, and respond proportionately;

5. make informed, independent best-interest decisions with the context of a DoLS assessment; effectively assess risk in complex situations and use analysis to make proportionate decisions.

(Community Care: Practice Standards for BIA 22/03/2013 accessed 21/10/2013 at **www. communitycare.co.uk/practice-standards-for-best-interests-assessors-launched)**

The six assessments

These six assessment are described in Schedule A1 Part 3 and are known as the 'qualifying requirements' which cover: age, mental health, mental capacity, best interests, eligibility and no refusals. All of these must be met otherwise the assessment under DoLS cannot proceed. A minimum of two people must carry out the process so now let us now examine just what each of these requirements mean, who carries this out and what form needs to be used. Although there is no legal requirement to use these forms, to help consistency and good practice this would seem to be a good idea that would help to alleviate concerns of different practices of recording evidence exists across the country.

Age
The person must be 18 years or older. This is determined by anyone who is eligible to carry out a best interests assessment using Form 5 or 10.

Mental health

The mental health assessment needs to be carried out by either a doctor who is s.12 approved or by a doctor with a minimum of three years' specialist experience in the diagnosis or treatment of mental disorder using Form 6.

Mental capacity

The person's mental capacity needs to be assessed by an approved doctor or a best interest assessor. The test of capacity was covered earlier in this chapter and must be in accordance with section 1-3 of the MCA using Form 7.

Best interests

Should be assessed by an AMHP, social worker, nurse, and occupational therapist providing that they have a minimum of two years' post-qualifying experience and have completed Best Interest Assessment training. Form 10 should be used.

Eligibility

To be assessed the person must of course fit the criteria and be deemed as eligible. This is set out in detail in Schedule 1A which although complex basically means that a person would be ineligible if they are already subject to detention under the MHA 1983 or a community treatment order, leave of absence or guardianship. In addition the person is ineligible if the main reason for detention is treatment in a mental hospital.

No refusals

This can be carried out by anyone who is eligible to do best interests assessment. Use Form 8. This rather odd element is drafted to see if a deprivation of liberty would conflict with advance direction or in other words to put the person in a similar position as someone who has capacity to refuse consent to the proposed action. Form 8 should be used.

BEST PRACTICE

Julie Jones is a 53-year-old woman with a diagnosis of learning disabilities, anxiety and schizophrenia. She has been an in-patient of an NHS community hospital for people with learning disabilities for nine months following a breakdown of her previous home circumstances. The hospital has been trying to manage Julie's slowly deteriorating behaviour which they say has necessitated more and more restrictions and restrain which have also interfered with her daily life. The hospital has identified the situation such that it may represent a deprivation of liberty.

At this point the hospital has referred the matter to the Supervisory Body who are the Local Authority in accordance with Schedule A1 of the Mental Capacity Act and following changes made in April 2013. This will invoke the use of the DoLS procedure and as this is not urgent the operation of a standard authorisation process which means that there is up to 28 days in which to complete the process.

The first stage would be to plan the process and initially to arrange for the Eligibility assessment *to be carried out if you are not an AMHP and for the* Mental health assessment *to be carried out and logically a s.12 doctor, using Form 6, could carry both of these out. This is important to plan early in the stage to avoid delay.*

The Age assessment *is completed using Form 5 and is for you to establish if the person is over 18 years (or will be once the process is complete). Usually this is not difficult and in Julie's case the medical records will confirm her age. An important point to note here is that although the MCA applies to persons over 16 years the DoLS only applies to those who are over 18.*

A doctor or a BIA can carry out the Mental capacity assessment. *This is carried out using a checklist approach, which is described in Chapter 4 and 5 of the MCA Code of Practice. Basically if the person lacks capacity the process continues but if they are on the balance of probabilities able to make their own decisions the process stops. Capacity must be 'decision specific', which means that it is about this time and this decision in particular. This should be made irrespective of appearance or behaviour. In this case the judgement is that Julie Jones does lack capacity. It is helpful to work through a checklist to make sure that it is a lack of capacity rather than a chaotic lifestyle or decisions, which you might think are unwise.*

The Age assessment *is completed using Form 5 and it was possible to confirm Julie's age is over 18 years and therefore the legislation applies to her. If the age isn't known you would have needed to estimate the age although this is very uncommon. If Julie had not been 18 years or would not have reached this age within the time limits use alternatives such as the Mental Health Act 1983 or the Children Act 1989.*

The No refusals assessment *needs to be established to see if there are any advanced decisions of lasting power of attorney for any decisions that might conflict with the deprivation of liberty that is being assessed.*

Having worked through the previous tests the final assessment is to carry out on Form 10 a Best interest assessment, *the process of which will help you to form a view about whether a deprivation of liberty is taking place, if it is in the best interest of the person and if yes if it is to be lawfully authorised. Arguably this is the most important stage and allows the decision to be evidenced and if appropriate to attach conditions. In Julie's case it could be argued that the DoLS timescale should be four months, which would give sufficient time for her social, care team to find her accommodation other than the hospital that would be more suitable.*

Resources

The *Mental Capacity Act 2005 Code of Practice* and *Making Decisions – A guide for people who work in health and social care* (OPG 603). Both of these are available to download for free from **www.publicguardian.gov.uk**

Best interests

It is a fundamental principle that any act or decision made for or on behalf of a person who lacks capacity is made in his or her best interests. This means that account will have been taken of the medical and non-medical effects and the overall welfare interests of the patient and the possible impact on the family. Section 4 of the MCA sets out the approach that must be used and just what must be taken into account when a best interest assessment must be carried out.

There will be best interest assessors (BIAs) who will be trained by the providers of AMHP training, and there will be mental health assessors (MHAs) who will undertake training provided by the Royal College of Psychiatrists.

Advance directions

Under the MCA ss.24–26, an adult while capable, may refuse medical treatment that would otherwise be provided to him in the future, when he had become incapable. This is now known as an advance direction (it was previously known as either an advance directive or a living will). If when the person has become incapable, the treatment in question would sustain his life, his refusal will only be binding if it is in writing and complies with other MCA formalities. In this way a person might refuse medical treatment that would have been given compulsorily under the MHA 1983. However, it might have some use in mental health care – for example, to prevent mental treatment being given to an informal, incapable patient (whose care would otherwise be given to him under the MCA) or in the case of a detained patient to prevent treatment being given to him for something other than mental disorder).

Court of Protection and the Public Guardian

Where an adult lacks capacity in relation to his health care or social care or his property or financial affairs, it is possible that the Court of Protection could make an order in that regard or appoint a deputy to make decisions on the person's behalf. The Court can only make an order to deprive an incapable person of their liberty if the requirements of the MCA 2005 Sch. 1 are met. The gateway to the Court of protection is through the Office of the Public Guardian.

Independent mental capacity advocates (IMCAs)

In most instances when problems arise with family, friends and communities provide a network of support for people. When people lose capacity this may become quite a challenge and when faced with major life-changing decisions they may need representation and support beyond that friends or family can offer. Thus the Mental Capacity Act (MCA) introduced the role of Independent Mental Capacity Advocates (IMCAs) on 1 April 2007 (October for Wales) and the statutory requirement to provide a specialist advocacy service for a specified group. This is a new and important safeguard for people who lack capacity and who have no one, other than paid staff, to support them.

The word 'advocate' originates from the Latin *advocatus*, meaning legal witness or counsellor. This is different from the role that IMCAs will play as they are described as *non-instructed advocacy*, as they are not taking instructions from the patient who benefits from their service. This is logical as the patient is deemed not to have capacity and therefore would find it difficult to instruct an advocate.

The IMCA is not a decision maker as such but the decision maker will need to take into account the information that is provided by the IMCA. Each local authority in England and each local health board in Wales provide an IMCA service. The role of the IMCA is set out in the MCA Code of Practice Chapter 10 as:

> *The purpose of the IMCA service is to help particularly vulnerable people who lack the capacity to make important decisions about serious medical treatment and changes of accommodation, and who have no family or friends that it would be appropriate to consult about those decisions. IMCAs will work with and support people who lack capacity, and represent their views to those who are working out their best interests.*

(p.178)

The important feature of this role is that it is one of advocacy and support with limited power to challenge or veto decisions made by the relevant authority. This really is a role in which the influencing skills of the IMCA will be important to represent the person who lacks capacity.

Where a person who lacks capacity and is without friends or relatives with whom to consult, decision-makers in local authorities, NHS trusts and care homes have a duty to consult with an IMCA. A person may be referred to the IMCA service if:

- they lack the capacity to make a decision;
- this decision involves changes to their long-term accommodation, e.g. under after-care,
- s.117 1983 MHA;
- they need serious medical treatment, e.g. surgery;
- they are subject to a care review and no one else is available to be consulted;
- they are in need of protection as a vulnerable adult whether or not family, friends or others are involved.

In practice IMCA clients will include those who are unconscious, have dementia, serious physical and/or mental health problems as well as end-of-life decisions.

The duties of the IMCA

There are a number of different roles that IMCAs take when supporting and representing people who may be subject to DoLS. These are set out in Section 39 of the amended MCA 2005. It is important to be clear as to which role the IMCA is taking, the roles are summarised as:

- Section 39A IMCAs are instructed when there is an assessment in response to a request for a standard authorisation, or a concern about a potentially unauthorised deprivation of liberty.

- Section 39C IMCAs cover the role of the relevant person's representative when there is a gap between appointments.

- Section 39D IMCAs support the person, or their representative when a standard authorisation is in place.

- The DoLS extended the role of IMCAs. Before DoLS the role related to decisions about accommodation, serious medical treatment, care reviews and safeguarding adults. IMCAs are instructed by the relevant local authority of NHS to undertake one of these roles. It could be advantageous for the service user if the IMCA took on more than one role but before they can do this, a specific instruction is needed by the relevant body.

(SCIE guide no 41, 2011)

Interface with other legislation, policy and procedures (see SCIE guide no 41, 2011, p. 47)

The Mental Capacity Act sits alongside other legislation, which you may need to be aware of the obligations under them. These would include:

- Care Standards Act 2000;

- Data Protection Act 1998;

- Disability Discrimination Act 1995;

- Mental Health Act 1983;

- National Service and Community Care Act 1990.

A more detailed look at these is beyond the remit of this book but you will no doubt realise that there is an abundance of information both in legal texts and online. However it is necessary to examine the interface between the MCA and the MHA. When the MCA became law it created in the words of Richard Jones, the author of one of the definitive reference books on mental health law, '...a recipe for confusion which will inevitably result in inconsistent practice' (Jones, 2012).

Choice of legislation

The Code of Practice to the MCA is helpful if you need to consider which of the two main acts should be used (although the Code's default is to use the MCA with the rationale that it offers a less restrictive alternative to the MHA). Brown et al. summarise the legal points well and the following is a summary of the key points that they make (Brown et al., 2009, p.120):

- The outcome of an assessment of a person's capacity will determine which Act or provision may be used lawfully.

- The MHA allows for informal and compulsory admission to hospital and treatment of mental disorder.

- The MCA allows for care and or treatment if it is in the best interests of people who lack capacity at that time but the MCA cannot be used to detain anyone.

- Some provisions of the MCA and the MHA can be used together but if the person is detained under the MHA, the MCA does not apply to treatment with the exception of ECT.

- All persons who are detained have a right to challenge this detention under law.

The MCA and children and young people

There is an overlap for children and young people aged 16–17 years between the Mental Capacity Act and the Children Act. Most of the provisions of the MCA do apply to young people and the MCA Code of Practice gives guidance on what to do in these circumstances. The person also needs to be over 18 years to make a living will and an advance decision to refuse certain treatments. DoLS only apply to people 18+ years.

CHAPTER SUMMARY

This chapter has introduced you to the complex area of law and the inevitable responsibilities that are placed upon professionals. To deprive someone of their liberty is so serious that legal safeguards are essential. The operation of Mental Tribunals is of paramount importance to the person concerned as well as reflecting on the professional capabilities of the professionals involved. The writing of an SCR is an important aspect of this and often not done well.

The role of professionals who have a key role to play in the operation of the Mental Capacity Act has been looked at in depth and through the case study you have covered one of the main processes through which people can be assessed under the DoLS. Although some of the roles are specialised, it is essential that all social workers understand the basic provisions of the Mental Health Act and the Mental Capacity Act and their corresponding Codes of Practice. Remember that all law is experimental and subject to interpretation and change – it is your responsibility as a professional to keep up to date.

FURTHER READING

Part 1

Fennell, P. (2007) *Mental Health: The new law.* Bristol: Jordan Publishing.

This is an excellent reference book. If you are interested in becoming an AMHP this is a key text for you study. For the Mental Health Act 2007 itself, see:

Department of Health (2008) *Mental Health Act 1983 Draft Reference Guide to the Mental Health Act 1983 as amended by the Mental Health Act 2007.* Can be downloaded (beware: over 300 pages) from **www.dh.gov.uk/publications**

For the hungry statistician, your first port of call should be the **Information Centre for Social Care.** They provide an annual publication, which summarises information about people detained under the 1983 Mental Health Act in NHS facilities, including high-security psychiatric hospitals, and independent hospitals. It includes figures for the period 1996–97 to 2006–07. Their web address is: **www.ic.nhs. Uk/statistics-and-data-collections/mental-health/mental-health-act/in-patients**

For a detailed and thorough understanding of mental capacity turn to **Brown, R., Barber, P. and Martin, D. (2009)** *The Mental Capacity Act 2005* (Second edition). Exeter: Learning Matters (Post-Qualifying Services).

For further information about social circumstances reports read **Curran, C., Golightley, M. and Fennell, P.** (2014) *Social Circumstances Reports for Mental Health Tribunals*, **Legal Action** Part 1 and Part 2 to be published March 2014.

Part 2

A must read for those who want more about DoLS is the excellent SCIE report *Deprivation of Liberty Standards: putting them into practice,* published October 2013 and available online from **www.scie.org.uk**

Office of the Public Guardian (2013) *Making Decisions: a guide for people who work in health and social care.*

The Mental Capacity Act OPG603 – another excellent assistance for you to read and consider. The DoLS Code of Practice 35 is an invaluable guide to help your understanding of the roles and responsibilities that are created by these safeguards.

IMCA and paid relevant person's representative roles in the **Mental Capacity Act Deprivation of Liberty Safeguards Guide 41**(2011) can be read at: **www.scie.org.uk/publications/guides/guide41/files/guide41.pdf**

Hargreaves, R. (2010) Briefing Paper 1 – Deprivation of Liberty Safeguards: an initial review of implementation at : **www.mentalhealthalliance.org/resources/DoLS**

WEBSITES

Note that the nature of the web often means that information needs checking carefully to make sure that it is the latest version.

Free downloads of two articles on the SCR can be requested from the institutional repository at the University of Lincoln using **http://eprints.lincoln.ac.uk/4349/** for Part 1 and **http://eprints.lincoln.ac.uk/4350/** for Part 2. When changes are made items are achieved until the most recent version is available.

Alternatively this can be accessed through a very useful website **www.hempsons.co.uk/news/hempsons-in-print/article/mental-health-tribunals-legal-action-journal/b2016582f5/?tx_ttnews[backPid]=579**

Chapter 5

Working with vulnerable people: mental health in children and adolescents

There is always one moment in childhood when the door opens and lets the future in.

Graham Greene (1940)

Introduction

In this chapter you will consider the kind of issues and knowledge that social workers need in order to carry out effective work with children and adolescents who have poor mental health. This will help you to understand the nature of these mental health problems and disorders and how to respond to them. Later on, the focus is on working with adolescents who are dealing with the problems of eating disorders, self-harm, dissociative disorder and depression. First you should consider the policy context and history.

Providing quality mental health services for children and young people has been a preoccupation of government. Policies in relation to children and young people have come and gone over the last decade and include (but not limited to):

2003 **Every Child Matters** which set out a framework for reform of children's services, including Children's Trusts and established five outcomes of being healthy, staying safe, enjoying and achieving, making a positive contribution and achieving economic wellbeing. The 2004 **Children Act** provided the legal backing for these and the five outcomes became almost a mantra for those of us in social work or education.

2004 saw the introduction of the **National Service Framework for Children, Young People and Maternity Services (NSF)** and set out 11 specific standards, included among which was Standard 9 – The mental health and psychological wellbeing of children and young people.

2008 was the publishing of the first **Children's Plan**. **The first Targeted Mental Health in Schools (TaMHS).**

2010 the **National Advisory Council for Children's Mental Health and Psychological Wellbeing** produced its first annual report. Also the age appropriate environment for young people detained under the Mental Health Act took effect (S131A).

Coalition government comes to power.

2011 The National Advisory Council produces its final report. The new mental health strategy is launched – **No Health Without Mental Health** – with the core theme of localism running throughout and sets out the six outcomes:

1. More people will have good mental health.

2. More people with mental health problems will recover.

3. More people with mental health problems will have good physical health.

4. More people will have a positive experience of care and support.

5. Fewer people will suffer avoidable harm.

6. Fewer people will experience stigma and discrimination.

Access to psychological therapies, the IAPT program for children and young people is introduced in a four-year plan of action in which the government commits £32 million to promote.

The **Me and My Schools project** was commissioned to examine how schools can help children and young people with mental health problems. (Report published in November 2011.)

2012 **Children and Young People's Health Outcomes Strategy** provided a forum to consult with stakeholders and reported back in 2012 with a sub-group report on mental health.

2013 Government responds to the report with the following:

- A commitment to do everything they can to improve the health of children and young people.

- Establishes the **Children and Young People's Health Outcomes Board**.

- Sets up a new **Children and Young People's Health Outcomes Forum** to provide ongoing expertise in child health.

- **Improving Children and Young People's Health Outcomes**: a system-wide response that follows on from the Forums set up in 2012.

Irrespective of the numerous policies and the shifts in direction the one theme that clearly stands out is that the emotional wellbeing of children and young people is as important as their physical health and a crucial factor in determining future health. Failing to deal effectively with emotional and mental disorders early on creates significant personal, social and economic costs. The presence of mental illness during childhood is one of the indicators of significant mental health problems during adulthood.

Some 'facts' (No Health Without Mental Health, 2011)

- One in ten children aged between 5 and 16 years has a mental health problem, and many continue to have mental health problems into adulthood.

- Half of those with lifetime mental health problems first experience symptoms by the age of 14, and three-quarters before their mid-20s.

- Self-harming in young people is not uncommon (10–13% of 15–16 year olds have self-harmed).

What social workers need to know to work effectively with children and adolescents

Social work with children and adolescents has until recently received little attention. However the government has endorsed the need for community and specialist services for this important group. Social workers have the skills necessary to work effectively with adolescents and to be key workers in multi-disciplinary settings.

There are many approaches that social workers and others use, some more effective than others. All have behind them a set of assumptions that raise issues for you, the service user and their carers. For example when working with an adolescent who displays behaviour associated with depression, is the adolescent the primary client or is it the worried parent? Working with the adolescent to help them to articulate their needs may be at odds with what their family want and believe should happen. A child may be bottling up feelings because they inwardly feel that to open up is to risk alienation of the family, yet it may be in their interests to express these feelings.

As a social worker you need to understand what the various mental disorders are in order that you can work alongside other professionals as well as undertaking direct work yourself. This is a complex area and you need to resist making simplistic assessments of complex situations and playing the role of amateur psychiatrist. Where your strengths lie is in using an empowering approach when you can work with people to help them discover explanations that they understand and ways of intervening that actually work for them. The real experts are the service users who have experienced for themselves the impact of mental disorder.

You could be working with children, adolescents and families as part of a team or approach or in your own right. The kind of problems that you could be working with can be categorised as follows:

Under 5s

- communication problems;
- sleeping difficulties;
- unusually strong or long-lasting tantrums;
- children who are suffering anxieties after major trauma or major life events such as divorce or separation of parents.

School-age but pre-adolescent children

- hyperactive problems;
- bed-wetting or soiling;
- relationship problems;
- behavioural problems at home or school;
- school refusal problems.

Adolescents

- eating disorders;
- behavioural problems;
- anxiety states;
- self-harm;
- depression;
- substance abuse.

Of course, before social workers get involved these problems and disorders must be perceived as either dysfunctional or disruptive and therefore it is essential to determine if this behaviour is within 'normal' or acceptable limits. Being in a position to do this requires that you have an understanding of the usual progression of children and adolescents and some knowledge of the kind of mental health problems and mental disorders that young people face. There are some disorders that are more closely associated with children and adolescents, even though they may also occur in adults.

Definitions of mental health in the context of adolescent development

Chapter 2 covered the main elements that make up a diagnosis of mental disorder and help us to appreciate mental health problems. It is worth revisiting this in the context of children and adolescents as there is a view held by many people that what we see as mental health problems are, in effect, simply signs of growing up that all of us have experience of. In other words if these problems are normal for adolescents the chances are that the young people will grow out of them and therefore we should intervene only as a last resort. The other view is that we should intervene earlier with relatively minor mental health problems to try to arrest them before they develop into something more serious. As a social worker you need to be clear about where you stand in this respect, as much of our work is at the crossover point between these views.

Adolescence is a period of development in our lives that is characterised by massive learning and assimilation of ideas as well as having to become a social being learning all the social mores. Writing about adolescence and the life course Crawford and Walker suggest that:

> ... it is the critical process of the development of self, the search for identity and the development of relationships, for example with friends, and the changing nature of relationships, for example with families, that are a central feature of this period of an individual's life.

> (Crawford and Walker, 2003, p.70)

It can be an intense time with significant pressures put on young people to perform at school and college and to reach developmental milestones. For some it can be the lack of opportunity and the disinterest of others in them that causes feelings of social exclusion and isolation. At the same time these pressures can produce stress, which as we have seen is one of the key intervening variables in the probable cause of mental health problems and onset of disorder (Chapter 2 provides more detail).

This needs to be put alongside on the one hand the popular view, often seen in the media, that adolescents are becoming more and more troublesome, while on the other hand is the romantic view of childhood innocence. Of course neither of these views is totally accurate and they illustrate the ambivalent attitude often shown by adults and the community at large towards adolescents.

Some Key Facts

Young Minds is a leading mental health charity focused as the name suggests on children and young people's mental health and it has produced some interesting statistics about mental illness and children and young people:

- *1 in 10 children and young people aged 5–16 suffer from a diagnosable disorder – that is around three children in every class.*

- *Between 1 in every 12 and 1 in 15 children and young people deliberately self-harm.*

- *There has been a big increase in the number of young people being admitted to hospital because of self-harm. Over the last ten years this figure has increased by 68%.*

- *More than half of all adults with mental health problems were diagnosed in childhood. Less than half were treated appropriately at the time.*

- *Nearly 80,000 children and young people suffer from severe depression.*

- *Over 8,000 children aged under 10 years old suffer from severe depression.*

- *72% of children in care have behavioural or emotional problems – these are some of the most vulnerable people in our society.*

- *95% of imprisoned young offenders have a mental health disorder. Many of them are struggling with more than one disorder.*

- *The number of young people aged 15–16 with depression nearly doubled between the 1980s and the 2000s.*

- *The proportion of young people aged 15–16 with a conduct disorder more than doubled between 1974 and 1999.* (YoungMinds at **http://www.youngminds.org. uk/training_services/policy/mental_health_statistics**)

Mental health problems and disorders in children and adolescents

One of the challenges to us is to understand the nature and extent of mental health problems and mental disorder that children and adolescents experience. These UK statistics can be compared with a 1999 study in the USA that showed that almost 21% of US children and adolescents aged between 9 and 17 had a diagnosable mental health or addictive problem and that for the more serious mental disorder the figure was 11%. The World Health Organisation predicts that there will be a significant increase in psychiatric disorders among children and adolescents that will place such disorders as one of the five most serious causes of death and disability among children (National Institute of Mental Health, 2003).

Good mental health is more than the absence of mental illness and the Mental Health Foundation (1999) suggested that mentally healthy children and adolescents would be those who can:

- develop psychologically, emotionally, creatively, intellectually and physically;

- sustain mutually satisfying relationships with others;

- use and enjoy solitude;

- become aware of others and empathise with them;

- play and learn;

- develop a sense of right and wrong;

- deal with problems and setbacks from time to time.

These development indicators are important for you to understand as they set the context within which you will develop your practice as a social worker, but of course they also require interpretation and reference to any previous history of mental health problems before considering someone's mental health. Equally valid is to get the young person's view of their mental health.

ACTIVITY **5.1**

Think back to your childhood and adolescence and using the above list see how well you managed to meet these developmental goals. How many of the above proved at some time in your development to be problematic? What constitutes 'normal' difficulties and what constitutes development that is not normal? Who is it that decides about this? Is it possible that you met the entire list but still had mental health problems?

Of course different people will have had different experiences and some of those will be determined by your gender, ethnicity, family circumstances and structural reasons like poverty.

Some young people who have experienced mental health problems and disorder believe that these lists do not cover all that is necessary for positive mental health.

Don't lose sight of the reality that it is adults who have determined what is satisfactory or not satisfactory about child and adolescent mental health. Walker points out that there is little evidence of young people having been consulted about their mental health problems. Consequently it is possible that what adults may want from children may well be at odds with what the young people wish for themselves.

(Walker, 2003)

Common mental health disorders

Although mental disorder can affect people of all ages there are some aspects that are more usually associated with certain age groups. Some of the more common mental disorders and mental health problems for adolescents are set out below.

Depressive disorders

These include major depression, bipolar and adjustment disorder that adversely affect the mood, energy and general social functioning of the young person. Most adolescents from time to time suffer from mood swings, depression and periods of hyperactivity, but the presence of these depressive disorders is distinguished from these by the duration of the symptoms and the extent that it interferes with everyday life.

There is a growing belief that a small minority of young people show signs of depressive disorders much earlier than has previously been thought and that this may occur during childhood. Depression often affects males and females differently but with both it is often difficult to uncover whether they are unhappy or depressed. The line between this unhappiness, which is short term, and the longer-term nature of depression is quite difficult to draw. Learning how to do this is down to experience and recognising some of the key signs.

The points at which concerns are raised relate to the extent of the behaviours and their intensity. For instance going into your bedroom for short periods and playing loud music is all part of being an adolescent, but going into your room, locking the door and refusing to have meals or to talk with the family is a point of concern if this lasts more than a few hours. This is a matter of degree and intensity and needs to be compared with previous behaviours.

Depressive disorders are closely associated with an increased risk of suicidal behaviour as the adolescent enters the post-15 years phase. One of the problems that clinicians face in making a diagnosis is that the *Diagnostic and Statistical Manual for Mental Disorders*, one of two psychiatric reference texts, uses criteria that are adult orientated rather than specific to adolescents or children. It is not that these criteria are incorrect but rather that they may be too narrow to cover adolescent behaviour (Pollack, 1999, p.320).

Once a decision has been made to intervene, medication and other talking treatments are indicated and often combined. Both counselling and cognitive behaviour therapy have proved to be effective when working with young people. Medication is often used although this needs to be carefully monitored as much less is known about the effect of this medication on children compared to adults. Indeed some medications, like some of the selective serotonin reuptake inhibitors (SSRIs) which are used extensively with adults, are not licensed for use on people under the age of 18 years as a result of considerable concern about possible side effects.

Hyperkinetic disorders or attention deficit hyperactivity disorder

Hyperkinetic disorder is the term used by British and European physicians when diagnosing attention deficit hyperactivity disorder/attention deficit disorder which it is claimed affects about 4% of the children and adolescents in the USA and a smaller but increasing percentage in the UK, estimated to be about 1%. In part this is as a result of psychiatrists in the UK adopting the more liberal diagnosis that is used in the USA. Signs include impaired functioning in situations where concentration is expected including classrooms and small group meetings. This can also manifest itself with impulsive behaviours and poor levels of functioning in relation to friends.

Interventions can either be medication, often Ritalin, or intensive behaviour modification or in some cases both. Ritalin is a psychostimulant and is from the same family as 'speed'. Although you would expect stimulants to make hyperactive young people more active it does in fact have the opposite effect for most young people.

Stimulant medication works for a short time and has the effect of helping the young person to concentrate and to work better at school as well as at home. Considerable gains in school performance and social ability have been reported. This medication works better when parent(s) are encouraged to provide practical and emotional support for their child. Stimulants are probably overused in the USA and underused in the UK and this medication is prescription only. Unfortunately in the USA and increasingly in the UK it is reported that young people sell this medication to their classmates as it also acts as an appetite suppressant. Young people may also 'save up' their medication and take a lot at once to get the 'buzz'. Where stimulants have not worked, doctors will often prescribe non-stimulant medication such as imipramine, fluoxetine or clonidine.

Social workers can provide behaviour management, counselling and psychotherapy. Children and young people will inevitably experience low self-esteem and will be challenging to engage with in any meaningful way. Often parental attention is craved for, even when it is negative, and parents may need your help to learn how to reward positive behaviours and to ignore the negative behaviour. Children with hyperkinetic disorder benefit from being rewarded as much as anyone else even though their extreme behaviour can be especially difficult and demanding. This approach may be as effective as prescribing medication.

It is important that you work with not only the young person and their family but also the school so that everyone is aware of what the intervention is and their role in the treatment plan. Disruptive young people can develop expertise in manipulation and the art of playing off one party against the other.

Dissociative disorders

This condition affects a person's sense of who they are and the extent that they engage with reality. The result can be a feeling of being 'disconnected' from their social world. Everyone can feel this way from time to time; for example long-distance runners sometimes experience a 'high' as they float through a marathon, which could be considered similar. A similar experience can also occur as a result of the side effects of drugs or alcohol.

As you can imagine a diagnosis of dissociative disorder is controversial. However, despite this it is likely that this disorder is much more common than previously thought. The diagnosis is often reached only after a series of several earlier misdiagnoses that can include borderline personality disorder and schizophrenia. The most complex of all of the dissociative disorders is known as dissociative identity disorder (DID) or multiple personality disorder in which the person experiences different personalities and often with an overlay of depression, severe mood swings, memory loss, anxiety and panic attacks.

The cause of this range of disorders is unclear but thought to include severe abuse in childhood and the lack of meaningful adult relationships that provide love and comfort. It is almost like the child or adolescent has had to be too self-reliant before they are capable of being so and has forgotten how to switch back to being a child. These disorders are diagnosed using some reliable tools such as the Dissociative Experiences Scale (DES) and the Structured Clinical Interview (SCID-D); a professional who is trained in this assessment tool must administer these. As with all mental disorders the cultural context needs to be uppermost in our minds when making such a diagnosis.

Social workers may work with people who have this disorder by providing information about self-help groups and by working with the person using a range of person-centred approaches. Self-help is often effective as are the various self-help groups and websites that exist (listed at the end of this chapter).

Self-harm

Self-harm, or self-mutilation, has been estimated to affect as many as one in ten teenagers and is the intentional infliction of harm upon themselves and YoungMinds in 2011 estimated that in England '100,000 children and young people could be hosptialised due to self-harm by 2020'; of course it is always difficult to rely on statistics more especially those looking so far ahead. These estimates were based on figures that Liberal Democrat MP Jo Swinson asked in a parliamentary question and showed 'that over the last decade inpatient admissions for young people have increased by 68% due to self-harm and that in 2010 inpatient admissions for under 25s increased by 10% due to self-harm and amongst females under 25 there was a 77% increase in inpatient admissions due to self-harm' (YoungMinds, 2011).

Self-harm often begins in teenage years and presents a considerable challenge to carers and professionals alike. It can be associated with other mental health disorders so it would not be a surprise to find that people who self-injure themselves experience depression, anxiety or panic attacks.

Self-injury is more common in prisons and 'care facilities' probably as a result of the difficulties that the young person is having in coming to terms with institutional life and social workers should be aware of this and be responsive to the young person. Self-harming behaviour is usually a private matter and it is unlikely, especially in the early stages, that help will be sought from a professional.

When trying to understand self-harm we need to think about why it is that most people do not deliberately injure themselves, in fact we have an inbuilt resistance to getting hurt or injured. One compelling idea is that we have a 'safety catch' that provides automatic protection against pain but self-harming involves at least temporally switching this catch to the off position (Tantam and Husband, 2009). We can all remember situations where we have been really scared of doing something but once we have done it the scariness becomes less and less and can turn into fun.

In the case of self-harm the safety catch is usually kept on by a powerful combination of fear and disgust whereas the factors that can lessen the strength of the safety-catch include:

- Impulsivity – the kind of person that we are.
- Intoxication – the impact that drugs and alcohol can have in dulling the senses.
- Habituation – the self-talk that justifies self-harming as an acceptable set of behaviours.
- Social norms and influence – being in an environment where this behaviour is socially or culturally acceptable.

If the concept of a safety catch has merit then we need to consider what triggers the release of this catch in the hope that by understanding this we will be in a position to at least understand why people self-injure themselves and through this be able to help them. Tantam and Husband (2009) write about emotional triggers that include feelings of powerlessness, suffering, resentment and fear – all the type of feelings that many of us but especially teenagers find hard to express.

There are a variety of reasons as to why people would do this including self-punishment, to gain feelings of control, clearing their mind, expressing their psychological turmoil physically, seeking attention/manipulating others, and the adrenaline rush that the body naturally releases during these actions. Self-harm, when practised frequently, can esca-late and become psychologically as well as physically addictive. The need to experience more severe harm in order to alleviate emotional pain and to attain an adrenaline rush is similar to the way that a drug addict would use increasing amounts of a drug in order to feel the 'high' they initially felt. Due to this a reliance on self-harm may develop which is difficult to stop. It is important for them to form a new coping strategy to replace this addictive habit.

LGBT people are more likely to self-harm than straight people. Self-harm is a warning sign that a young person has experienced abuse, particularly sexual abuse.

National Self-Harm Network

0800 622 6000 (7pm–11pm) **www.nshn.co.ukinfo@nshn.co.uk**, offers support and information for people who self-harm. Here you will find information about what is self-harm, misconceptions about self-harm, how family and friends can support someone who is self-harming and a helpline and online support.

Eating disorders

Eating disorders involve serious disturbances of the 'normal' eating pattern, and an obsessive concentration on body size and diet. These disorders can be seen on a contin-uum from minimal intervention in the community through to life threatening conditions that require specialist residential services. Eating disorders are real, treatable mental dis-orders that can cause considerable distress to those who are experiencing the effects of the disorder and to their carers. (This is used as a case study later in this chapter.)

Social work interventions

Interventions range from working with families to individual work. You need to reflect on some of the value and ethical issues when working with young people. In Chapter 1 the issue of who is the primary client was raised which showed some potential conflicts of interest. In particular the dilemma of conformity with parental demands may be at the expense of the young person's emergent sense of self. Equally, working in an empowering way with the young person may be liberating for them but at the cost of their relationship with their parents and families.

Intervention can take many forms but family support is often the most common and most effective. This can consist of working with the family as a whole and/or working with individuals in the family. The thrust of government policy epitomised in the *Quality Protects* child and family consultation paper (DoH, 1999) is that early intervention by offering advice and support to parents will eventually reduce the number of people who at a young age are diagnosed as having a mental disorder (Walker, 2002).

The choice of intervention is considerable and it is important that services reflect service user needs rather than being resource driven. The following table sets out some of the main interventions that social workers and others might use, depending upon individual circumstances.

Type of intervention	Key aspects
Cognitive behaviour therapy (CBT)	Cognitive techniques challenging negative thoughts and behavioural techniques used to relieve maladaptive thoughts, beliefs and behaviours
Systemic and family therapy	Works on relationships within the family and patterns of interaction between the members
Interpersonal therapy (IPT)	Focuses on the interpersonal relationships of the service user; helps to improve communication patterns and how people relate to one another
Psycho-educational methods	This takes various forms and includes work with service users and families to help them to understand the nature of their disorder and how to promote their mental health
Counselling	Can take many different forms – usually one-to-one and gives the individual the opportunity to develop their understandings of their reactions to events

(Adapted from *Treatment Choice in Psychological Therapies and Counselling*. DoH, 2001)

There are occasions when a combination of interventions works; for example CBT and IPT are effective when working with people who are depressed and help to reduce the symptoms of depression (see above).

The National Service Framework for Children in 2003 restated that children's mental health is everyone's business and set the aim of developing a comprehensive CAMHS service. This saw a rapid growth in training programmes to increase the capacity of the workforce at all levels to be able to cope with these increased expectations.

One of the major features of this approach is the Common Assessment Framework (CAF), which will be an assessment process that is used by all the workers in children's services. This is a simplified pre-assessment checklist, a process for carrying out these assessments: a standardised form to record and to share with others.

Lesbian, gay, bisexual and trans people

This section explores what social workers should do in order to make a difference in the lives of children and young people who are LGBT in general and adolescents in particular and who experience mental health problems. Although public respect of the LGBT community has undoubtedly increased over the last decade there is much more that needs to done. In England, with the repeal of Section 28, a law that banned so-called 'promotion' of LGBT 'lifestyle' in schools, and with advent of same-sex marriage legalisation, there are many ways that LGBT people are still treated unequally in our society. LGBT people remain disproportionately more likely to experience mental health problems then non-LGBT people.

To be clear, LGBT people are being discussed in this book not because of a belief that being lesbian, gay, bisexual or transgender is a mental health problem. To the contrary, it is being discussed because society has a homophobia, biphobia and transphobia problem that can have devastating impacts on the wellbeing of LGBT people. For example, a young person who is LGBT may fear family rejection, community exclusion, school bullying, street harassment, and abuse for openly acknowledging their gender and sexual orientation. Such actions can result in high levels of stress and as we know this is an intervening variable often associated with mental health problems.

Key terms

In order to present a culturally competent approach to LGBT people we must first, as practitioners, reflect on our own gender and sexuality as well as the culture in which our profession is situated. We will discuss this using a Queer Theory approach, which takes a critical examination of the gender and sexual norms that are reinforced through day-to-day interactions, the media, government and capitalism. First let's look at some key concepts and terms:

- Gender.
- Sex.
- Gender binary.
- Transgender.
- Genderqueer.
- Cisgender.
- Cisnormativity.
- Sexual orientation.
- Queer.
- Heteronormativity.
- Intersex.
- Intersectionality.

How many of these terms were you already aware of? How can a lack of practitioner knowledge about these terms create barriers to LGBT support? Why not select a couple of these terms and search the web for further information.

Experiences of mental health services

You may know that being homosexual was once classified as a mental disorder in the DSM. This pathologising of identity had the consequence of damaging interfamilial relationships and in some cases treatment that was designed to elicit 'cure' of the affected individual. Thank goodness times have changed but this does further illustrate the dangers for us as social workers of accepting what turned out to be a pseudo-scientific approach. In the current DSM, men who dress in 'women's clothing' remain potentially diagnosable, despite the fact that many women in what would be considered traditionally 'men's clothing' (i.e. trousers) have no such equivalent diagnosis. Children who do not abide by gender norms are likewise often provided with 'treatment' to reinforce gender normative behaviours and can be diagnosed with a mental health issue. So a young boy in makeup, skirts and nail polish may be given 'corrective-therapy' whereas a young girl doing the same is likely given praise.

LGBT people report that what they want is support that affirms their identities and experiences, rather then pathologises them. In so doing we must inform ourselves to deliver services that are relevant and accessible to LGBT people. Practitioners should be aware of how oppression impacts on mental health, housing access, employment opportunities, and heightened risks of experiencing violence.

Best practice example: working with transgender people

Many of us grew up being told that we are a girl or a boy and that we must dress, act and fulfill social roles accordingly. Some of you may have never doubted whether or not you feel that you are supposed to be a girl, or a boy. Transgender people are people who were assigned as male or female at birth and have an internal sense of gender that doesn't match this.

Some transgender people refer to themselves as a 'transman', or a 'transwoman', which means they should be treated as male and female, respectively. Some transgender people choose to identify as 'male' or 'female' only and without the prefix of 'trans'. Others may not identify as either male or female, and may come under a wide range of gender expressions. A transgender person may be lesbian, gay, bisexual, or heterosexual.

Some transgender people seek to 'transition'. Transitioning is a broad term that can include a person changing their name, attire, pronoun, and in some cases accessing hormones or medical procedures. A transgender person should be treated according to the gender they say that they are. Under the 2004 Gender Recognition Act trans people have gained legal recognition for their acquired gender, including a new birth certificate. It follows that it is illegal and degrading to ask intrusive questions about people's genitalia, surgery, or Gender Recognition Certificate in order to ascertain what gender they are. The 2010 Equality Act treats gender identity as a protected charac-teristic alongside eight other grounds and brings with it rights of public sector equal-ity and protection, in law at least, against discrimination. If you are unsure about how to relate to a 'transperson' the recommendation is to ask: 'What name would you prefer for me to use?'; 'Would you like for me to refer to you by "he", "she", "they" or something else?'; 'How do you define your gender'? You may also want to ask how they would like for you to refer to them when sharing notes with other practitioners – remember the service user may not be 'out' as transgender to every-one else, and it is illegal to disclose this information without permission.

It is important when supporting a transgender person that their being transgender is not seen as 'the issue' at hand. Be person-led in your approach. Only discuss their being transgender when it is relevant. If a person is seeking support for grief, they may not feel that being transgender plays a large role in this, it may be unhelpful to talk about a person's transgender status when the conversation focus should be about mourning loss. However, a transgender person who has lost a trans community member to hate crime or suicide may find it very relevant to discuss how transphobia impacts on their life and that of their community.

Transgender people may be interested in transgender and LGBT specific services avail-able to them. It is recommended to have LGBT and transgender specific resources available, for example, having a list of helplines and support groups that are in your local area. Also don't forget that these issues are not confined to children and adoles-cents, LGBT inclusive practice is important throughout service user's lifespan.

To read more about this area try the excellent book

Fish, J. (2012) *Social Work and Lesbian, Gay, Bisexual and Trans People: making a dif-ference.* Bristol: The Policy Press.

and

Hines, S. (2007) *TransForming Gender: Transgender practices of identity intimacy and care.* Bristol: The Policy Press.

You may want to make a note of the following (great places to work once qualified or to undertake a placement)

National Organisations:

Mermaids – www.mermaidsuk.org.uk

Family and individual support for teenagers and children with gender identity issues.

Stonewall – www.stonewall.org.uk/

Working for equality and justice for lesbians, gay men and bisexuals.

Gendered Intelligence – genderedintelligence.co.uk/

Understanding gender diversity in creative ways.

Albert Kennedy Trust – www.akt.org.uk/

Supports lesbian, gay, bisexual and trans homeless young people in crisis.

Broken Rainbow – www.brokenrainbow.org.uk

Providing the National Helpline for lesbian, gay, bisexual and trans people experiencing domestic violence: 0300 999 5428 (LGBT).

Imaan – www.imaan.org.uk

Support for LGBT Muslims.

Terrence Higgins Trust – www.tht.org.uk/sexual-health/Sex-and-relationships/ Sexuality-_and_-gender

Sexual health for LGBT people.

Queer Youth Network – http://lgbtyouth.org/

Online discussion forum for LGBT youth.

Services for children and adolescents

Child and Adolescent Mental Health Services are organised into four tiers of service. These are important for professionals who are involved in this area of work to understand as is the connection between the various organisations who provide services for children and adolescents. This structure is set out below and is adapted from the *CAMHS Handbook* (DoH, 1995).

First tier: primary care

This is the level at which interventions are made by GPs, health visitors, school nurses, teachers and social workers. The distinguishing feature of this tier is that it is generally provided by non-specialists who can work with children and adolescents in ways that are non-stigmatising but still open up the possibility of early recognition of mental distress. This level of service is usually provided at a local level wherever the professional works.

Second tier

This level of service is provided by a uni-professional group, which includes clinical child psychologists, educational psychologists, child psychiatrists, community child nurses and social workers. This tier offers specialist training for first tier workers and consultation for professionals and their families as well as outreach services where specialist services are not indicated and they also offer assessment for tiers three and four. This level of service is provided at a small number of locations within the community.

Third tier

At this level of service this is a specialist service for people who have more severe and complex disorders. This is typically a multi-disciplinary team often working in a community child mental health clinic or outpatient service. This will include social workers, child and adolescent psychiatrists, clinical psychologists, occupational therapists and art and music therapists.

Fourth tier

This offers access through assessment to child psychiatric services including day units and residential units including in-hospital services for children and adolescents who are in need of highly specialised services. These include services for people who are severely mentally ill or who are at risk of serious self-harm or suicide. These are the most specialised of services and likely to be provided at a supra-region level as not all districts can resource this level of expertise.

Although this is the structure currently in use the National Advisory Council is proposing that this tiered approach is replaced by a simpler and more defined three levels of service that are described as *universal, targeted or specialist* (NAC, 2010). It is still unclear when this change will occur.

Compulsory admission to hospital

For the purposes of the MHA a child is anyone who is under the age of 18 years. There are no lower age limits (other than guardianship, which may not be used for a child under the age of 16 years). Children and young people may be admitted to a psychiatric facility in one of four ways:

1. Informally with their consent providing they are deemed to be 'Gillick competent' – this is a matter for the treating doctor to determine.

2. Informally through the agreement of the parent or someone who has parental responsibility if they are incapable of consent, but note that the 'Deprivation of Liberty Safeguards' under the MCA 2005 do not apply to those under the age of 18 years. Children who are under 16, but admission would not amount to a deprivation of liberty, can be admitted under MCA 2005 ss.5 and 6.

3. Under s.25 of the Children Act 1989 should be used if the primary reason is to deprive the child or young person of liberty for their own safety or for the safety of others (rather than the treatment of mental disorder).

4. Under the MHA Part 2 or Part 3 would be used if the primary reason is the treatment of mental disorder and they meet other requirements. Note once subject to this order the child could be placed in secure accommodation without a court order because this is sufficient power to detain them.

(Fennell, 2007)

The guiding principles are basically the same as for adults, with the note that 'any intervention should be the least restrictive and the least stigmatising option consistent with effective care and treatment but also should result in the least possible separation from family, carer, friends and community or interruption of their education as is consistent with their well-being' (Draft Code of Practice, p.212).

Children and young people have special needs and it is important that such expertise is mobilised. There is a requirement that at an assessment of a young person, one of the professionals who is involved should be a specialist in CAMHS. This could be an AMHP or a clinician.

If a child or young person is admitted to hospital he/she should be accommodated in what is referred to as 'age-appropriate facilities', which would exclude admission to an adult ward. This is in fact a limited duty under s.131A MHA 1983 to have accommodation that is suitable having regard to his/her age (subject to needs). Providers should consult a CAMHS specialist to make sure that this duty is met. There are now restrictions on the informal admission of 16–17 year olds to the effect that if the young person has capacity and does not consent to admission to hospital, then this cannot be overruled by the consent of the person who has parental responsibility for the young person.

Children and adolescents who are socially excluded

This group has been identified for specific attention by the government which has set targets for socially excluded young people and provided funding for specific projects. Such children and young people could be from asylum seeker families, or refugees who may have been witness to considerable trauma, both of which can magnify their experiences of isolation and exclusion in the UK. Although common-sense tells us that such experiences must cause stress and that this can result in mental disorder there is no conclusive evidence. What we do know is that the stress of living in a family at the edges of society is in itself likely to cause mental health problems for members of the family including children. This will include the effects of physical and emotional abuse that may result from continual pressure and the isolation of parents. The impact of racism upon children and such families is under-researched but again it is likely that this is a compounding factor, which results in mental disorder for some young people.

Black and minority ethnic children are, like some of their adult counterparts, over-represented in the mental health system. They may have suffered from developmental delay and other problems that are not of their making but may be a result of social exclusions and racism.

ACTIVITY 5.2

Imagine that you are have arranged for a young girl aged 14 to visit you at the office to discuss mental health problems that she has talked about with her teacher. Write down what factors you think are crucial to helping to build up a good relationship with her, e.g. provide a suitable setting.

The ideas that you might have come up with would include:

- *Having a suitable setting that is welcoming, private, safe, secure, has few distractions, materials to draw or write with, comfortable seating alongside each other.*

- *Plan the session and read the previous session's notes.*

- *Boundaries need to be set, identifying what will be discussed and what will not be discussed.*

- *Keeping an open mind is important to allow you to gather valid evidence with the young person acting as your guide.*

- *Listening and reflecting are basic interviewing skills for you to use to get as full a picture as possible about the young person's life and the analysis of their situation.*

- *Empathy and intuition, trying to walk in the young person's shoes, will help you to understand what is going on for the young person and how she assesses her situation.*

- *Safety: always ensure that you are not left exposed to allegations about your conduct which may mean that you need to leave the room door open or interview with another colleague.*

Engaging and communicating with adolescents

Adolescents may be referred to you by their parent, teacher, or be seen by you as a result of other work that you are doing with the family. Adolescents are usually difficult to engage in any form of therapeutic work. Many professionals think that specialist mental health services only reach about 20% of adolescents who need these services. For all those adolescents who do reach out and engage there will be many more who will see you once or twice, and that will be enough and they disappear off your files. Of course it could be that even brief interventions can work and it can also be that a positive experience at least sets up the possibility of a return by the adolescent at some later stage.

However, it may be important to help adolescents and young people early on in their lives to develop mechanisms that enable them to resolve difficulties that may adversely affect their mental health in later life. If adolescence is a time of transition between life stages it is also a time in which learning occurs about how to deal with the inevitable problems that life throws up. Faulty learning at this stage can result in longer-term mental health problems.

ACTIVITY **5.3**

From your experience write down what you think are some of the 'life events' that adolescents may have to deal with when growing up.

We can all draw upon our personal experiences and those of our friends when we went through this stage in our development. Ann Weal (1999) draws upon research to list some of these events which include:

(Continued)

(Continued)

- *conflict in the family;*

- *experience of being in care;*

- *poor development of verbal, literacy and academic skills;*

- *unmet emotional needs.*

To which you probably could have added bullying at school, peer pressure to look good, go to parties, have a boyfriend/girlfriend, have sex, not to have sex, etc. The list quickly grows and with it the potential for tension between competing demands.

Eating disorders

'Eating disorder' is a generic term that includes anorexia nervosa, bulimia and compulsive over-eating. These can develop into serious and often complex disorders that cause considerable anxiety and distress for the young person and their families. MIND estimate that one in 100 women in the UK between the ages of 15 and 30 experiences anorexia. Male representation is much smaller although growing in prevalence (National Institute of Mental Health, 2001). Eating disorder is ranked as the third most chronic illness in female adolescents (USA brief notes on the mental health of children and adolescents, October 2003).

Anorexia nervosa affects teenagers, usually girls, who are typically perfectionists and have the potential to do well at school but sometimes they can be over achieving or nearly failing in school. They may have the additional diagnosis of obsessive compulsive disorder (OCD). They will typically have low self-esteem and may believe that they are fat even in the face of seemingly overwhelming evidence that they are emaciated. Many teens experience a fleeting sense of control when refusing food and may enjoy the food battleground that has been created with parents or carers.

Bulimia has different symptoms from anorexia and the teenager will typically binge on huge quantities of food and later eliminate the food through the use of powerful laxatives or self-induced vomiting. Such binges can be alternated with periods of diet. It can be hard for parents and others to discover bulimia as people become quite clever in concealing this condition as the adolescent may be of average weight (due to bingeing and then dieting). Also purging can occur with any food intake which, although strictly would not be classified as bulimia, is included as an eating disorder not otherwise specific (EDNOS) or atypical eating disorder.

In diagnostic terms adolescents are usually considered separately from adults as the strict diagnostic criteria of the DSM IV may not be entirely applicable to adolescents. For example adolescence is a time when there is wide variability in weight, height and sexual maturation as well as cognitive development which may make this diagnostic tool unreliable. This can result in some adolescents who have anorexia nervosa going undiagnosed (Society for Adolescent Medicine position paper, 2000).

The treatment options depend upon the nature and development of the condition. Assessment needs to include clinical manifestations and social and psychological contexts. This is best carried out with an interdisciplinary team approach and may need to cover nutritional advice and counselling.

In a small number of instances there may need to be a period of hospitalisation followed by attendance at a day programme and a supported return to school or the community. The aim should be to provide a seamless transition from inpatient care to outpatient and to be person-centred.

What factors lie behind anorexia and other eating disorders?

A major study involving over 2,000 people in Australia has shown that those who previously dieted to a severe level were five times more likely to experience an eating disorder than those who dieted moderately. This led the research team to suggest that a safer way to control adolescent weight would be through an exercise programme and an educational input about diet and shape.

The connection between diet and the development of eating disorder is not made in every case. However:

> *every morning hundreds and thousands of women wake up worrying about whether it is going to be a 'good day' or a 'bad day' in relation to food. They feel remorse for what they ate yesterday and hope that they will have more control today.*

(Orbach, 1986, p.1)

Orbach suggests that eating disorders, in particular anorexia nervosa, have become metaphors for the way in which society attempts to shape our lives and in this case the bodies of women. In this scenario women find themselves having to mediate their passions and desires, often in a public way, to achieve what they perceive as the desired physical shape. Thus eating can become a ready-made battleground on which women regularly seek to starve themselves to get closer to the perceived perfection of the catwalk model.

While anorexia, bulimia and compulsive overeating do not affect all women, the issues about shape and the centrality of food to the female experience mean that the issues about eating and the realities of eating disorder can be seen as an extreme manifestation of the inner turmoil that many women feel in relation to their bodies. Thus Orbach suggests that the adolescent girl must learn to develop a split between her body and the development of herself and that the girl fantasises over the benefits that might come her way with a slimmer body. This can be hard for men to appreciate and, especially, to understand the messages that men give out to women about their desirability.

There is no overall theory that can explain how this condition begins but there is agreement that stressful events can be seen as an intervening variable that might trigger off mental disorder (see Chapter 2 for a more detailed explanation). However, eating disorders are not just about shape and diet, they can occur as the adolescent attempts to get control over their lives or to punish themselves for events often out of their control but for which they feel very guilty. The onset of the condition is sometimes linked to previous sexual abuse or other significant physical or psychological trauma. It may also be that the young person is making an unconscious attempt to slow down or even prevent her body developing during adolescence and an attempt to avoid sexualisation of her body. All these ideas are interesting and of course relevant to our study and if you are going to work in this area or experience this condition yourself you will need to read more.

Although there is dispute over the actual cause of eating disorder there are some common factors. The most important of these is the way in which the person needs to feel in control of at least a part of their lives. People with eating disorders often feel that controlling their eating in such a severe manner is the only way that they can control their lives. Those on the outside, paradoxically, may see this as the ultimate expression of someone who has actually lost control of their lives.

This is primarily a condition that affects women, but the number of boys and men affected by eating disorders is on the increase. At present they account for about 10% of identified eating disorders (Neustatter, 2003). It is quite possible that as society becomes more obsessed with the human shape, men are beginning to feel the pressure of being the ideal shape and that this striving for the unobtainable perfect body produces casualties on the way. Anorexia is more common in trans people, especially transwomen trying to lose weight to appear 'more feminine'.

The social work response

Listening and trying to understand the person's experience and not jumping to conclusions that are not supported by evidence is key. People who experience this distress are often smart, self-critical and competitive people. They can be very able to discuss all aspects of their condition without getting down to the personal reasons about why they are that way and how they can begin to get a better balance in their lives.

CASE STUDY

Lisa's story

This case study is based on the personal and professional experience of young people who I know and have worked with. I have altered the case to disguise their identities but without losing the essential features. It may surprise you to look at young people's narratives and to see just how many similarities there are between them.

For Lisa the arrival of anorexia was like the arrival of a person who lived inside her head and who had an alternative view of the world. This voice spoke deep down inside and said what to eat and what not to eat. At the age of 14 this voice came to live with Lisa. She couldn't remember the exact day but can recall that the effect was that this voice was struggling for control over her eating habits.

Lisa is a smart young woman who was self-critical and into alternative politics and protests.

At first Lisa was strong and felt that she was able to control the voice and argue with it when the instruction was to eat nothing. The struggle with the voice became very tiring. What do you say to those around you about the arrival of a voice? She was experiencing a degree of dissociation and in particular dissociative identity disorder with each identity assuming control at various times.

The easiest approach was to avoid eating with other people and to have a commitment to a harsh vegetarian diet. These combined made it more acceptable not to eat regular meals. She switched from school meals to a packed lunch, which she threw away. Gradually people around her, her family and friends, began to notice and it became a battleground at meal times. No one understood the struggle that was going on for her with her voice that she thought of as being evil but which no one else knew about. She wore several layers of loose-fitting clothes, which hid her weight loss. These strategies concealed the loss of weight and the reality that she had become very skinny.

As Lisa began to lose weight and her skin and hair showed signs of poor nutrition she took the bold step of seeking help from the school and a referral was made to the educational psychologist. At this point she was in a poor frame of mind, worn out by the battles with the voice and lacking in energy. One night she took a large quantity of anti-depressants, paracetamol and anything else that was to hand, all washed down with a large quantity of vodka.

Discovered by her mother she was admitted to the accident and emergency unit and given life-saving treatment. The following day she was transferred to a specialist unit. Here she was able to have her eating carefully monitored and to receive specialist input from the team, which included a child and adolescent psychiatrist, psychologist and social worker. She went to a 'group' where she learnt that others had experienced similar situations and also had voices that sought to control their food intake and kept telling them that they were overweight.

The support of the other young people in the unit was especially helpful and contrasted with the general lack of understanding in the world outside of the unit. The unit brought together her immediate family once a week for a Saturday group where attempts were made to help the family recognise the difficulties that Lisa faced and the family's role in this. It was here that the family learnt not to keep on at Lisa for not eating and that trying to persuade her to put on weight was making the situation worse rather than better. It

(Continued)

139

(Continued)

was difficult for the family to accept that Lisa was not doing this to hurt the family but was engaged in a struggle that was hers alone and that the most helpful approach was for them to listen to Lisa, try to understand and to offer their support.

Over a period of a few weeks Lisa got into a position where she pushed the voice into the background and learned some techniques that helped her to keep it there. She was also prescribed anti-depressants and a mood stabiliser from her psychiatrist. Every morning she was weighed and her weight gains recorded. Any loss meant reduction in privileges and closer attention being paid to her diet, a process that she resented but deep down knew helped.

Today Lisa continues to have mental health problems but the eating component of her disorder is at least under control and the eating voice has subsided. Now that she has a more understanding family she can draw some strength from this support although she realises that outside of a small circle there are few people who will understand what she has been through.

Early intervention

Early warning signs are important to recognise and early intervention may well have prevented Lisa's later hospitalisation. Tiers one and two are usually the first point of service and late referrals can be put down to families and friends mistaking signs of mental health stress as 'natural' or 'normal behaviour' for adolescents. Among the general signs are the following:

Emotional signs

- sad or anxious without apparent reason and for unusually long periods of time;
- constant concern about appearance;
- feelings of worthlessness.

Behavioural signs
Look for behaviour that has changed recently or causes comment by others:

- poor concentration;
- nightmares/insomnia;
- loss in women of menstrual cycle;
- sudden and unexplained significant weight loss;
- alcohol or drug misuse including laxatives;
- self-induced vomiting;
- concern about diet and calorie counting;

- wants to be alone;

- over-exercising;

- light-headedness and/or fainting;

- evidence of purging.

Recognising early signs

All the above need to be put into the context that change is a 'normal' part of adolescence. Equally, families may be reluctant to seek help, fearing the negative effects of labelling of their child. Ignoring early signs of mental health problems in children and young people can have detrimental long-term effects. Early intervention will mean working at the preventative level with young people before their mental health problems become mental disorder.

In Lisa's case several factors were noted as set out below:

- Her parents had divorced and there was still considerable acrimony between them. Lisa was often caught up in the middle of these battles and having to make judgements about competing demands.

- Several friends had noticed that she was more and more withdrawn and spent less time in company and more time on her own listening with headphones to her music.

- She was becoming more obsessive about a number of things including dietary needs, likes and dislikes.

- Her schoolwork had fallen well below her previous level and certainly below what the teachers thought that she was capable of achieving (in some cases there is a sudden dramatic increase in grades).

Tier one services could have helped at this stage and avoided the risk of stigma and labelling that a late referral to the specialist might bring. Increasingly social workers are being located in schools and colleges, which can help mobilise an early response. The Connexions service has personal advisors often located in schools who can also provide easy access to services at levels one and two.

ACTIVITY 5.4

You are a social worker placed in a secondary school. Lisa's friends have come to see you as they are concerned about her. What action would you take? Think about this using the 'assessment framework'. Would you:

(Continued)

(Continued)

- *talk to Lisa?*

- *talk to Lisa's parents?*

- *talk to Lisa's teachers and others at the school?*

COMMENT

Depending upon what happened with your preliminary assessment it might be appropriate to refer Lisa for supportive counselling and/or put her in touch with a self-help group. It may be wise to check out how these work as there have been cases where some groups are used to check out and exchange dieting tips though this is often an undercover activity and therefore hard to recognise. There are also numerous websites that are great sources of information and which Lisa might want to visit. You should check out what your local CAMHS website is.

Interventions

There are two types of interventions, those that are called **psychological therapies** and those that are **clinical interventions** and these are summarised below. Like work with adults the emphasis needs to be on provision of a multi-disciplinary approach that is evidence based. Before using any form of intervention you should check the evidence to see what works best in what situation and what skill level is needed to engage with service users.

Psychotherapy

Psychotherapy focuses upon our inner world and through a process of insight development, usually on a one-to-one basis, helps to develop a greater awareness of the nature of an eating disorder and to understand possible causes. Through this understanding people are in a better position to get control over their eating disorder. The theoretical position of this intervention is based in the work of Freud, Klein and Piaget. This form of intervention is usually undertaken by psychologists, psychiatrists or a counsellor and can cover all tiers of CAMHS although usually this intervention is at tiers one and two.

Cognitive behaviour therapy

This focuses not on the inner world of the young person but on the actual behaviours. Here the cause is less important than the manifestation of the behaviours and there is a belief that the causes may not be able to be changed but the behaviours can be altered. The therapist or social worker will work with the person to help them to identify negative and counter-productive thoughts and replace them with a more positive frame of mind. Usually used at tiers one and two.

Dialectical behaviour therapy

This is an approach that is derived from CBT in which the 'therapist' seeks to work with the young person both accepting and validating their feelings while trying to help them to see that some feelings and behaviours are not working for them and then to help them to identify better alternatives. The combination of CBT techniques of emotion regulation and reality testing with concepts of distress tolerance, acceptance and mindful awareness can be effective and owes much to the adoption of Buddhist meditative practice.

Psycho-social intervention

This draws upon theoretical positions that are founded in the social sciences and see the person in a social context allowing for intervention that recognises the importance of empowering interventions. Here social workers play a crucial part, as they are unique in being able to work with the service user. By so doing they can understand what is happening to the service user and to recognise and intervene to provide access to self-help groups, advocacy, etc. Usually a tiers one and two intervention.

Alternative therapies

These are widely available, often in local community centres or in specialist agencies like MIND, but are increasingly also available for inpatient treatment. These therapies help the person to find alternative ways of expressing themselves through movement, dance, art, poetry and music. There are also a number of self-help texts that some service users report as being very helpful (see further reading). Usually a tier one service but can be across all tiers.

Inpatient

In an extreme case of eating disorder the person's health can be at serious risk as weight loss and nutritional imbalances reach life-threatening proportions. This is tiers three and four and requires a whole-team approach if the condition is to be reversed before long-lasting damage occurs. Specialist clinics are available which may operate under specific therapeutic regimes. Any programme of treatment should form part of a person's agreed care programme (Code of Practice, 18, p. 87) and all treatments should follow a full discussion of the form that the treatment will take, and how and when it will be reviewed.

In some cases young people may be 'force fed' under the Mental Health Act (1983) and social workers may be required to sign the legal forms as a person not connected directly with the treatment of the patient but one who knows that patient's circumstances.

Irrespective of the theoretical approach that you have chosen to use it is important to work with service users as people just like you and me and whom deserve the very best social work that you are able to deliver. Avoiding treating people as if all they are is a set of symptoms and a diagnosis and look behind these to find the 'real person'.

Stress busting tips

Managing stressful distractions when trying to study

One of the main problems when trying to get down to serious study is the inner dialogue, which goes on in our minds and keeps playing messages like 'I cannot do this' or 'I am not clever enough' or 'I'd rather do – well anything but this'. Avoidance of hard work like learning seems to be part of a common human condition but using some principles from cognitive therapy can help you to alter these inner conversations and by so doing reduce the impact of stress.

How to turn down the inner voice volume

- Close your eyes.

- Listen to all those negative words until they become clear.

- Imagine this is like a radio – reach out and turn the volume up.

- Listen and make sure that the voices in your head do become louder.

- ENJOY YOUR CONTROL.

- Reach out and turn down the volume – notice how the voices go lower.

- Continue until the sounds become distant and resemble the gentle murmur of the ocean on a still day.

- The sound is still there only now you cannot even make out the words.

- Practise this technique so that managing these internal conversations becomes easier each time that you use this technique.

This method of stress busting requires practice and can be effective for you. With care and skill it can also be used when working with adolescents who are struggling to engage with school.

CHAPTER SUMMARY

In this chapter you have read about some of the difficulties and issues that young people experience, that for some, develop into mental health problems. The point has been made that the emotional and mental wellbeing of young people is as important as their physical health and how they respond to such issues can be a positive or negative effect on their subsequent development as an adult. Social workers can often play an important role in a team approach to work with children and adolescents. Social workers have the skills and levels of understanding to be able to undertake direct work with children and adolescents. Best practice in social work includes being culturally competent, including being LGBT affirmative. In the chapter a variety of conditions were examined and in particular self-harm and eating disorders which both present challenges to services are examined.

FURTHER READING

Walker, S. (2003) *Social Work and Child and Adolescent Mental Health.* Lyme Regis: Russell House.

This is one of the few and certainly the best reads in this area. In this book you will find many of the ideas in this chapter covered in more depth. All chapters are good but Chapter 7 on socially inclusive practice is relevant to this area of work and pulls together the recent government ideas and gives out ideas for a broad ranging practice that works to combat the worst effects of social exclusion. For principles underlying assessment read chapter 3.

Smith, G. (2004) *Anorexia and Bulimia in the Family: One parent's practical guide to recovery.* Chichester: Wiley:

This is a practical guide, written by a parent whose daughter experienced anorexia, and is good reading as it combines practical advice with latest research.

Useful organisations

MIND – The mental health charity that provides a voice for people with mental health distress and disorder. It also has a range of fact sheets and publications that make essential reading for those who want more information about mental health. It also runs a number of supportive workshops and user groups. This could be your first port of call for alternative health care, information and/or support **www.mind.org.uk**

Dissociative disorder

Useful websites include:

www.dissociation.co.uk

A resource for professionals.

www.mosaicminds.org

A website that offers assistance for survivors of childhood trauma and has a particular focus on dissociative disorder.

www.ukssd.org

This is the UK society for the study of dissociation.

Eating disorders

Eating Disorders Association offers help and support for people who experience eating disorder. Young person's helpline: 01603 765050.

www.edauk.com

Overeaters Anonymous. Although based in Manchester this organisation runs local groups for compulsive overeaters. Tel: 07000 784985.

Pale Reflections is a popular website for adolescents who find the material accurate and informative. This is a USA site.

www.pale-reflections.com

Association for Dance Movement Therapy. Promotes dance therapy and can provide lists of locally based qualified therapists. Email enquiries to dance.voice@cableinet.co.uk

The Institute for Optimum Nutrition. Sells books, tapes and videos and can refer callers to nutritionists throughout the country. Tel: 020 8877 9993 Email allion@ion.ac.uk

The Mental Health Act Commission publishes a series of Guidance Notes among which is the technical and detailed Note No. 3 on *Guidance and Treatment of Anorexia Nervosa under the Mental Health Act 1983* which was published in August 1997. Tel: 0115 943 7100.

ADD/ADHD Family Support Group UK offers support for families. Tel: 01373 826045.

A great website is provided by the Royal College of Psychiatrists – **www.rcpsych.ac.uk** – which has information sheets that cover many of the topics in this chapter.

YoungMinds, 102–8 Clerkenwell Road, London EC1M 5SA. Tel: 020 7336 8445 **www.youngminds. org.uk** this provided the idea of a timeline of policy and for a fuller version than I have provided go to this site.

National Institute of Mental Health at **www.nimh.nih.gov/publicat/eatingdisorder.cfm**

National Institute of Mental Health (2001) *Eating Disorder: Facts about eating disorders and the search for solutions.*

A detailed booklet describing symptoms, causes, and treatment, with information on getting help and coping.

National Self-Harm Network 0800 622 6000 (7pm–11pm) **www.nshn.co.ukinfo@nshn.co.uk,** offers support and information for people who self-harm. Here you will find information about what is self-harm, misconceptions about self-harm, how family and friends can support someone who is self-harming and a helpline and online support.

Chapter 6

Working with vulnerable people: adults who are short-term service users

The liberty of the individual must be thus far limited; he must not make himself a nuisance to other people.

John Stuart Mill (1859)

ACHIEVING A SOCIAL WORK DEGREE

This chapter will help you to develop the following capabilities from the **Professional Capabilities Framework**:

- **Professionalism**
  Identify and behave as a professional social worker committed to professional development.

- **Values and ethics**
  Apply social work ethical principles and values to guide professional practice.

- **Diversity**
  Recognise diversity and apply anti-discriminatory and anti-oppressive principles in practice.

- **Rights, justice and economic wellbeing**
  Advance human rights and promote social justice and economic wellbeing.

- **Knowledge**
  Apply knowledge of social sciences, law and social work practice theory.

- **Intervention and skills**
  Use judgement and authority to intervene with individuals, families and communities to promote independence, provide support and prevent harm, neglect and abuse.

It will also introduce you to the following standards as set out in the 2008 social work subject benchmark statement:

5.1.3 Values and ethics.
5.1.5 The nature of social work practice.

Introduction

This chapter will help you to understand the impact that acute episodes of mental health issues can have for someone and to investigate just what your role as a social worker is at these times. It builds on the learning that has occurred during the previous chapters. The initial focus is on living with depression and helping to prevent suicide. The role of primary care teams and the need for effective liaison across a range of bodies will be examined. To some extent separating out acute need from the following chapter where chronic need is covered is artificial as often today's short-term or acute user moves to being a long-term or chronic user of services. Our starting point is to examine depression and in particular suicide.

A case example is used to show how social workers may need to work with a service user who is potentially suicidal. This highlights key areas such as community care and direct payments. Emphasis is placed in this chapter on assessment for services and the imaginative use of resources. This will cover how social workers can work with providers to provide 24-hour crisis support services.

Policy context

The statistics

Suicide is a major public health issue and is one of the major causes of death in England, Wales and Scotland accounting for approximately 15% of all deaths annually, although the exact numbers are unclear due in part to the reluctance sometimes of coroners to find a verdict of suicide. This is partly due to varying criteria but also out of respect for the families. Thus it is quite likely that this figure of 15% is an under-representation of the actual number of suicides. This means that every year about 6,000 people in England, Wales and Scotland kill themselves. In these statistics you will find that men outnumber women by almost 3:1 and in the UK, the age group with the highest rate is males between 40–44 years and for females 50–54 years (Samaritans, 2013).

Suicide reduction

The national suicide prevention strategy for England Our Healthier Nation (OHN) was launched in 2002 with a very ambitious aim of reducing deaths by suicide to 7.3 per 100,000. The most recent annual report of progress since the national suicide prevention strategy for England was published in 2010 based on data collected in 2007/8 and showed a fall in the overall rate of suicide amongst the general population aged 15+; at 9.8/100,000 these were the lowest recorded in this country, although the latest figures suggest that this rate has since risen to an overall figure of 10.4.

Surprisingly the amount of data on suicide is limited with information on ethnicity, social-economic status not routinely reported. There is also the potential for a distorting effect to occur if the population overall is small and this is the case for suicide in older people. This is also the reason why suicide in under 15 years is not reported as it is so small it could distort the overall rate. Consequently you need to use these statistics with caution.

What these statistics do not do is to explain why suicides occur and we are left to use conjecture that perhaps economic downturns and the resultant austerity measures have impacted on people's feeling of despair and helplessness. It makes sense to me but that is as far as one can go with these.

The government meanwhile has promised £1.5m to fund research that will explore what further steps could be taken to try and prevent suicides among those at highest risk. The strategy was launched so as to coincide with World Suicide Prevention Day in 2012. Already we can see attempts to block harmful suicide-related websites, focus upon mental health facilities and prisons as places where not only is the risk is high but the prospect of intervening is good. Of course if there was a simple solution it would have been found by now so bear in mind what the chair of the National Suicide Prevention Strategy Advisory Group, Professor Louis Appleby said: 'Suicide does not have one cause – many factors combine to produce an individual tragedy. Prevention must too be broad – communities, families and front-line services all have a vital role' (**www.the guardian.com./society/2012/sep/10/suicide-prevention-strategy**).

Assessment of people who pose a risk to themselves is a complex and difficult task whether they live in the community or are hospitalised. If they live in the community one of the goals will be to achieve a balance between providing good quality intervention and avoidance of unnecessary risks. Admission to hospital is used as an example to help you to understand when this is necessary.

The Confidential Inquiry

The **National Confidential Inquiry into Suicide and Homicide** is based at the University of Manchester and is commissioned by the Healthcare Quality Improvement Partnership (HQIP) on behalf of the NHS England, NHSSPS Northern Ireland, the Scottish Government, the Welsh Government, and the Channel Islands. The most recent report was in July 2013 and is replete with statistics and trends from all of the UK countries. Some of the trends that are relevant to this chapter are:

- Suicide by mental health patients (1,333 deaths in 2011 (England)) has risen, and although comparisons with previous years are difficult as a result of coding changes, still represents a true increase.

- There have been more suicides under home treatment or crisis resolution than under inpatient care (all countries). A substantial proportion of these deaths occur in patients who live alone or have refused treatment – home treatment may not be suitable for these patients without close supervision.

- Patient suicide is still frequently preceded by missed contact with services (England, Scotland and Wales) and in Northern Ireland the numbers of such cases increased during the report period. Northern Ireland is the only UK country not to introduce assertive outreach teams (or an equivalent) although in England these teams are in some places being reabsorbed into general Community Mental Health Teams (CMHTs).

- The effect of CTOs on patient suicide is unclear. CTO suicides may follow treatment refusal or loss of contact which they are designed to prevent, suggesting they could be applied more effectively (England, Wales, and Scotland).

The above findings have been extracted and adapted from the actual report and I recommend that you visit the website to see the context in which they are written. The National Confidential Inquiry into Suicide and Homicide can be accessed from: **www.bbmh.manchester.ac.uk/cmhr/research/centreforsuicideprevention/nci/reports/**

There are numerous survey findings over the last decade but a recurring theme is that the most common life event before suicide was the breakdown of a marriage or partnership, followed by: bereavement; physical illness and financial problems (adapted from Eldergill, 1998). Relevant to our case example is the finding that over half the people who had committed suicide had contact with the services the week prior to that event.

However it also has become clear that some groups are over-represented and that these have not been clearly identified. Of particular note is the suicide risk among Lesbian, Gay, Bisexual and Transgender people (LGBT), which is thought to be especially high. Organisations representing lesbian, gay and bisexual groups have expressed concern that the suicide prevention strategy did not address the perceived disproportionate levels of suicide and self-harm among these groups (particularly young gay men). In addition, a recent study examining the mental health and social wellbeing of LGB groups in England and Wales concluded that levels of substance-use disorders were higher in gay men and lesbians. Results also showed those gay men and lesbians reported more psychological distress than heterosexuals. For further information consult **www.nmhdu.org.uk/silo/files/ sha-letter-pacepdf-23rd-september-2009.pdf**

Elsewhere organisations have claimed that Black and Minority Ethnic (BME) women have become invisible to mainstream services and are absent from government policies and sponsored research. Their argument which is powerful is that equality and diversity issues are dealt with rather than addressing the more complex relationship between race and gender at the point where BME women intersect (*Safe and Sane*, 2011). For further information request a free copy of *Safe and Sane*, Hannah Siddiqui and Meena Patel Published by Southall Black Sisters Trust, 2010. **www.southall-blacksisters.org.uk/**

BEST PRACTICE

Southall Black Sisters run a project that responds to the needs of black and minority ethnic women who experience both domestic violence and mental health problems. This project has built upon over 30 years of work with women who have a wide range of mental health problems and most have contemplated suicide at lease once in their lives and many have attempted suicide and self-harm. Their experience suggests that South East Asian young women, often with no recorded previous history of mental health problems, are up to three times more likely to kill themselves than the general population.

In this context they established work that allowed BME women to be both safe and sane. Their own evaluation of the project shows reduced incidence of domestic violence and mental health problems (as indicated by low repeat victimisation) and a greater sense among the women of safety and wellbeing.

They use a holistic approach in what they have called the 'SBS model', which is a new 'hybrid' form of psychotherapy bringing together elements of individual counselling, psychotherapy with advocacy and practice advice. This rather eclectic yet effective approach is specifically geared towards the specific race and gender needs of BME women who often have complex needs with very few, if any, places to seek help.

We now make the move from policy to application and consider the case of Mr Skeffling (this is his preferred mode of address). This case is used throughout the remainder of this chapter to show how assessment and intervention can be made and what research and statute should inform the kind of decisions that you as the social worker would be making with the service user.

CASE STUDY

Phase one

Mr Skeffling lives with his wife in a remote country village. He is 68 years old and she is 69 and they have lived in the same area for the last 20 years or so. They have two children, both adults, who live in cities some 55 miles away. Mr Skeffling has become depressed and has been prescribed anti-depressants by his GP. Mrs Skeffling returned home after visiting her son for a couple of days to find her husband in a very distressed state. At first she was unsure if he had been drinking heavily but he eventually told her that he had taken a large amount of his medication all at once and washed it down with his favourite whisky. He said that he was 'absolutely fed up with life – it was all too much and he had had enough'. She called her doctor who made arrangements for Mr Skeffling to be admitted informally to the local psychiatric unit.

COMMENT

The admission to hospital was made in order to provide Mr Skeffling with an environment that could respond to the immediate risk and assess the next step. A referral is made to the community mental health team and as the social worker you visit first thing the following morning. By this time Mr Skeffling has settled and is feeling somewhat embarrassed by in his view 'all the fuss about nothing'. He knows that in the last few months he has been very down, isn't very happy with the diagnosis of depression but wants to go back home as soon as possible.

Depression and suicide

How common is mental disorder among older people? Depression in old age is far more common than many people think. Various estimates suggest that as many as one in four older people have symptoms of depression that require treatment with this rising with age so that 40% of those over 85 will have depression (National Mental Health, 2011). More women are affected than men. Other severe forms of mental disorder are also prevalent including of course the organic form known as dementia. When you consider that in England we are experiencing an ageing population, the actual number of older people with mental disorder is gradually rising. In 2008 there were 18.3 million people aged 60 and over in the UK, and it is estimated that by 2033 that those over 75 will increase from the present 4.8 million to 8.7 million and from 1.3 million to 3.3 million for those over 85.

If you work through these figures you will realise that we are talking big numbers and estimates of two million older people experiencing depression are not far short of reality. But can depression be linked to suicide? The obvious answer is yes, but this does need some careful examination before assuming that one necessarily leads to another. First the reality is that the highest suicide rate is found among elderly people and in particular those over 75. This is still the case even though the actual total number of people who successfully kill themselves has begun to fall in recent years.

General practitioners are at the front line when it comes to recognising depression in people. In the case of older people, depression can be overlooked if the GP wrongly thinks that older people are unlikely to be depressed and instead perhaps concentrates on physical problems. The co-morbity of mental illness and physical illness are becoming better understood and we recognise depression is more than seven times more common if you are an older person and have two or more chronic physical conditions. Depression increases the risk of coronary heart disease. Equally depression can follow major medical events and interventions such as cardiac bypass operations. This is now part of the new mental health strategy.

> *The second objective of the No Health without Mental Health strategy adds weight to intervention is more people with mental health problems will recover – and have a good quality of life – greater ability to manage their own lives, stronger sense of purpose, the skills they need for living and working, improved chances in education, better employment rates and a suitable and stable place to live.*

(2011, para. 3.16)

Identifying ways of differentiating depression from the usual effects of older age, which could include sleep disturbance; lowering of activity levels; lower libido and/or greater level of fatigue presents a challenge for practitioners. There are a number of specialist rating scales that help the professional recognise the symptoms of depression and make this task easier and more valid. These include the Geriatric Depression Scale (GDS) (Ulas and Connor, 1999). Like most disorders early recognition usually offers the best chance for good recovery.

Traditionally services are organised in tiers or levels with access to the higher tiers being through the referral system. Primary care is the first tier with services being provided by the GP and other professionals. The general principle is that people's mental health needs should be met at the lowest tier possible and this will involve other agencies such as social services and the voluntary sector. Localising services through Clincial Commissioning Groups are one of the policy intiatives that ought to bring more appropriate services nearer to where the demand is.

Social factors

CASE STUDY *continued*

After a week in hospital Mr Skeffling returns home agreeing to take the anti-depressant medication and to work with the team to develop the care plan into a more comprehensive one. As the social worker you will take on the role of care coordinator/key worker. This includes visiting him at his home.

After two interviews with the couple it is becoming clear that their relationship is not especially strong and that Mr Skeffling feels ignored and isolated. Whereas at one time he was a full-time farm worker he is now retired and on a fixed and modest retirement income. His best friend died last year, which has left him with a sense of despair.

What factors contribute to depression? The psychosocial model, suggested in Chapter 2, helps to identify possible factors and for Mr Skeffling in particular the importance of loss to him. His close friend and really only male friend in the last 20 years has been his near neighbour who died seven months ago. The two of them shared an interest in going to the nearby village pub in the neighbour's car and enjoyed the atmosphere and watching live football matches. Mr Skeffling has been once or twice since but felt very isolated and thought that everyone was looking at him. The only time that he gets out is to go shopping in the nearby town, which he finds uninteresting.

Although Mr and Mrs Skeffling have been married for a long time they appear to have got bored with each other's company and when together they frequently niggle at each other. He is critical of how his wife spends her time and their money while she complains that he is taking root in front of the television. Whereas his wife has a circle of female friends whom she meets twice a week in the church hall, Mr Skeffling doesn't have anyone to talk to or to confide in.

As a further complicating factor Mr Skeffling's car is playing up and will need major repairs or replacing soon. They both say that they cannot afford a new car or to spend a lot on the repair of their present one. Yet without the car they will be unable to go shopping or to make the odd trip to the town. Their children are adults who live quite a distance from them and only get to visit once a month at best and without a car the couple will not be able to go and see them.

CASE STUDY *continued*

The assessment of the situation that the couple find themselves in is starting to take shape. You should now see what factors you have identified as important from the above illustrative example and the notes afterwards.

COMMENT

The importance of loss as a significant factor in the onset of depression will probably be the first that you picked up. In this case it is a double hit as not only did Mr Skeffling lose his activity but also the only person with whom he appeared to have a close, confiding relationship.

Social work and suicide

Not all suicides are associated with mental disorder although the presence of a severe mental disorder increases the risk of suicide. It has been estimated that of the people who do commit suicide 90% experience mental disorder of some type and of these about 30% have expressed clear intent to kill themselves and 25% are psychiatric outpatients. This presents a real challenge to mental health teams. We now need to examine what factors need to be considered in Mr Skeffling's case.

Colin Pritchard describes various ways of estimating suicide risk and uses the Lettieri scale for older men which pinpoints the following key factors:

1. Recent serious loss.

2. Depression.

3. Element of anger or aggression in their behaviour.

4. Refusal to accept help.

5. Previous suicidal or self-harming history.

6. Failure in a major role of their lives.

(Adapted from Pritchard, 1995)

These represent what might be termed 'negative factors' and if you relate this to Mr Skeffling you can see that numbers 1, 2, 4 and 6 are present in varying degrees. This Lettieri scale is one of a number of measuring tools that assist in the prediction of suicide among the population. There are also several self-assessment scales that are in use. They vary in their clinical usefulness and the main use is to aid decision-making but not to replace it.

It is necessary to distinguish between risk of suicide in the short term and risk in the longer term. It has been estimated that about 2% of those who had one attempt will succeed within a year of the first attempt, with a particular risk occurring in the first three months (see Butler and Pritchard, 1983). The difficulty that social workers and other clinicians have is assessing just who are the people who fall into this category. This requires a balance between identifying those most likely to be at risk while not intervening unnecessarily with those who are considered to be a lesser risk.

An additional approach is to work with the service user to help identify with them the positive factors or the 'reasons for living'. This approach assumes that the service user will be able, with help, to identify reasons for their life and to be able to put these alongside the more negative attributes. This helps you to work with the service user to identify their strengths or assets rather than only weaknesses or deficits.

ACTIVITY **6.1**

Write down what you would consider to be the reasons for living that would be relevant for you and then write down what you think Mr Skeffling might say and compare the two.

COMMENT

I hope that you found plenty to put down for yourself. I think that Mr Skeffling would struggle a little with this and probably need prompting but he might list:

- *hope that life will change;*
- *love of his family;*
- *being scared of the act of suicide;*
- *moral objections about suicide;*
- *a view that suicide is a sign of weakness.*

(Adapted from Linehan, 1985 in Pritchard, 1995)

Working with people who have attempted suicide

The most important contribution that you can make as a social worker is to manage to work alongside your health colleagues to provide a joint approach yet retaining the essential and unique features of social work. A major concern when working with people who have attempted suicide is how or perhaps even if this should be discussed. There are many excellent texts about working with people who are at risk of suicide or serious self-harm.

In our case the psychiatrist at the unit will have carried out an assessment and this will have been discussed at the care planning meeting that will have taken place before discharge took place. The type of questions would include the following:

Questions about the incident itself:

- What was his intent?

- What is the relationship between his depression and this attempt?

- What is the risk at the present of a further attempt?

- What kind of help would he be willing to accept?

CASE STUDY *continued*

Mr Skeffling denies that this was a serious attempt. He has been suffering from mild to moderately severe depression for the last few months but also admitted that he has not been taking his medication regularly. No particular event led to the attempt but he describes it as a build up of events such as the death of his friend and the increased isolation that he feels. He is willing to work with the team to seek ways of improving his life. This would put him in the low risk category.

Questions about the degree of intent

- Was the attempt planned or impulsive?

- Did he know that he would be found soon after the attempt?

- What drugs were taken? How much alcohol was taken? Were there other drugs that were around but not taken?

- Was a suicide note left?

CASE STUDY *continued*

Mr Skeffling's attempt at suicide was not thought through and it appears impulsive. He used his prescription medication as the means of trying to 'end it all' and chose a time when his wife was out but also not long before he knew that she was going to return. No arrangements for following his death, suicide notes, or update of his will, were evident. These put the likelihood of suicide in the low to moderate category.

Assessment of current problems

- Relationship with family members.

- Financial status.

- Social networks, support isolation.

- General health.

- Use of alcohol or drugs.

The above is adapted from a number of guides to assessment (Butler and Pritchard, 1983; Eldergill, 1998; Pritchard, 1995).

According to Age UK, the number of 55 to 64 year olds living alone has increased by 50% since 1998. Social isolation is now thought to affect more than 1 million people in the UK, and the evidence that social isolation is a risk factor for dementia and shortens lifespan is becoming irrefutable. People can feel isolated and very much alone within dysfunctional relationships as well as being physically on their own. **(http://www.theguardian.com/social-care-network/2013/jul/11/reduce-social-isolation-declining-social-care-budgets)**

CASE STUDY *continued*

Mr Skeffling's relationship with his wife has worsened over the last few years and he has no other person in whom to confide. He is struggling to get by financially and in particular is really anxious about living where they do and being without a car. His wife has a strong network of friends but most of his have either died or left the area. He does drink at home by himself from time to time and when he does it is often to excess. He is not very optimistic about the future. This puts him in the moderate risk category.

COMMENT

The use of such assessment tools should only be undertaken by someone who is skilled and experienced in their application. They are in common use and different clinicians favour different tools. Eldergill has drawn together some of the research findings in this field and some of these are set out below.

Source	Research findings
J.H.J. Bancroft and P. Marsack, *British Journal of Psychiatry* (1977) 131, 394	The risk of completed suicide is increased where there is the presence of mental disorder and alcoholism.
A.R. Beisser and J.E. Blanchette, *Diseases of the Nervous System* (1961) XXII, 7, 365–9	The risk of another suicide attempt is most common within three months of the first attempt.
S. Ganzler et al., *Life-Threatening Behaviour* (1971) 1, 184–202	A significant link can be made between attempted suicide attempts and social deprivation.
N. Kreitman, *Parasuicide* (John Wiley, 1980)	1–2% of people who attempt suicide kill themselves within 12 months.

(Adapted from Eldergill, 1998, p.733)

All research should be treated in a critical manner but also needs to be carefully considered and referred to by professionals. This is how professionals continually develop, yet there is evidence that suggests that while medical practitioners may consult the research as a matter of course this is not the case with other professionals such as social workers.

Risk assessment

The evaluation of the above risk factors needs to be undertaken by a clinician who will weigh these up against the research. In the case of Mr Skeffling his behaviour appears to be more of a response to the present situation and discontent with his social isolation and financial situation than total despair with his life. Mrs Skeffling is on paper a viable carer but their relationship is difficult and more likely to be part of the problem rather than the solution. He has only recently seen the doctor for depression and at the time this was assessed as being mild. Since the initial emergency call-out Mr Skeffling appears to be less despairing and to have appreciated the opportunity to talk though his worries with someone who is outside of the family.

ACTIVITY **6.2**

Look back at the developing case of Mr Skeffling and jot down what you think are the risk factors. What role could Mrs Skeffling play in the situation?

Policy background

The late 1980s and the 1990s witnessed the move from a policy that was focused upon long-stay hospital care to one that focused upon the provision of services in the community. The closure of large psychiatric hospitals and their community replacements meant that health and social services in many instances had to learn to work together and this is still an ongoing process. This theme ran throughout many government policy documents with suitably aspirational titles like *Building Bridges* (DoH, 1998); *Partnerships in Action* (DoH, 1998); *Modernising Social Services* (1998); and *Modernising Mental Health Services* (see DoH, 2002).

Care in the community – expanding services to offer choice

The mental health service as it is evolving has the ideas of choice and localisation as central and defining features.

By offering service users choice they can be better matched to appropriate services depending upon their need. That present-day services are unresponsive, in many instances, to service user need is generally accepted but in order to have choice there would need to be an excess of supply over demand which seriously impacts on service efficiency. Thus services continually come up against the stark financial realities and it has proved difficult for services that are genuinely user-focused to be developed in times of austerity. To offer genuine choice means starting not with what services can be matched but what the service user needs. This requires innovation on the part of service providers and the imagination of those charged with assessment and planning (Onyett, 1992). It also means considerable resources need to be poured into making community care a positive choice that will enhance the lives of vulnerable people.

The key statute relating to care in the community is the National Health Service and Community Care Act 1990, which actually came into being in 1993. This Act has since been supplemented by The Carers (Recognition and Services Act) 1995, which introduced the right for carers to have an assessment of their needs made alongside the service user's assessment. The Community Care (Direct Payments) Act 1996 also enabled local authorities to provide cash for service users to enable them to purchase the kind of services that they want. The later HSCA 2001 made it a duty from April 2003 for local authorities not just to offer direct payments but extended the coverage to include people of any age. This has now developed into an approach called personalisation that SCIE in an excellent document describe as:

> *Personalisation means thinking about care and support services in an entirely different way. It means starting with the person as an individual with strengths, preferences and aspirations and means putting them at the centre of the process of identifying their needs and making choices about what, who, how and when they are supported to live their lives. It requires a significant transformation of adult social care so that all systems, processes, staff and services are geared up to put people first.*

(SCIE, 2010)

Personalisation key features

The most important aspect of personalisation means a new way of thinking about care and support services. Rather than starting from what we have been used to providing, the new approach means starting from where the service user is and determining the individual's strengths, preferences and aspirations. This sounds so easy but in practice it has needed lots of training in different localities just to help professionals grasp the central features.

The hope is that over time this will become the norm and will begin to break down the stigma of mental health and seriously reduce the extent of institutionalisation that is associated with mental health. This is a values-driven approach to mental health services and a transformation on a large scale. To achieve the objectives of policy, providers of services will need to engage positively with service users, carers and expert by experience. These are exciting times!

However, even with all these bold policy initiatives community care remains patchy and in many instances problematic.

CASE STUDY *continued*

Mr Skeffling has returned home and an assessment has been carried out to determine if he is eligible for community care services. It is quite clear that his wife, who is unable to drive, is unable and unwilling to take responsibility for her husband's wellbeing. She is very frightened that he might do something silly to himself.

Getting help depends first on having a Community Care Assessment that meets the 'eligibility criteria'. The assessment places service users into one of the following bands: critical, substantial, moderate or low. The assessment is a full one and may take time to organise and carry out but this does not prevent services from being provided or payments made until this occurs. Too often the assessment is about eligibility for existing services and how best they can be packaged to suit the service user instead of working with the service user to identify what would work well for them and carry out a genuine assessment of need. Any assessment ought to look not only at what is missing but also the strengths of the service user and their individual environment.

The criteria that are used may vary slightly from area to area but will include some of the following in order to be put into the critical band:

- significant health problems have developed or will develop;
- inability to carry out vital personal care or domestic routines;
- social support systems and relationships cannot or will not be sustained;
- family and other social roles and responsibilities cannot or will not be undertaken;
- engagement with vital formal support systems is not being maintained;
- serious risk of harm to self or others exists;
- inability to access community facilities.

CASE STUDY continued

From what you have read about Mr Skeffling use the above list to check out if he meets any of the criteria and the level of importance to him.

COMMENT

The extent that he meets the above is largely dependent upon how you see the situation. This is an important point for assessments need to conform with equal opportunities which means taking time and approaching the assessment with the service user and others (if appropriate). Work like this needs skill, patience and transparency and the assessment should be signed off by all interested parties.

In the above activity it is likely that he meets all of those criteria but the question is the extent to which these are seen as vital or significant. Allocating assessment to bands is the next step to decide if he is eligible for community care services. In our example Mr Skeffling may just about meet the social services eligibility criteria at least in the short term.

What services can be provided?

Services will be provided to people who are unable to perform one or more basic tasks of daily living where:

a. informal support (Mrs Skeffling) cannot be reasonably expected to provide them;

b. service users (or their carers) are at significant risk without the provision of such services; or

c. services are clearly aimed at increasing independence.

Services will be provided to:

a. meet essential personal, social and educational needs;

b. ensure that service users and/or carers are not left at significant risk;

c. support carers to continue in their caring role;

d. support people to continue living in the community through a programme of rehabilitation.

Most councils have set up a direct payment support service of some sort to help people purchase their own services and to assist them with the legal obligations of employing personal assistants and accounting for the money. The scheme was widely extended in April 2003, which has resulted in a large increase in take up. Local authorities now have a duty to offer direct payments.

Support and self-help

The scheme that came into being is Direct Payments (Community Care (Direct Payments) Act 1996) that allows service users who are disabled, including people who have mental disorder, to receive cash payments in place of services from social services. The intention is that they will support service users who wish to remain independent but the use has been very restricted (Robbins, 2004). This approach was built on the views of what service users want and it was apparent that they wanted:

> ... *Information, help with ordinary living, support with personal growth and development. They want well co-ordinated packages of treatment, and a plan that takes account of their aspirations for the future.*

> (Robbins, pp.2–3)

The Direct Payments scheme offers another alternative that could be very empowering for the service user. When it was originally launched it had age restrictions and close relatives could not be paid. Unsurprisingly take up was low and these restrictions were removed with the HSCA (2001) legislation. The recipient is also responsible for managing and accounting for the money, which in turn most likely will require assistance and/or training.

Check out on the internet what information your local social care provider gives to potential mental health users. Putting in the key words 'direct payments' into a search engine such as Google will give you lots of information. If you had a mental disorder would you know where to go to get information and once you have the information would you want to have these payments? Although you might be eligible, the thought of having to administer money yourself and to keep accurate and verifiable records may in themselves be a deterrent and turn you away from the direct payment solution. Most local authorities have websites for direct payments although these can be out of date.

Alternatives to traditional hospital-based services

Acute and crisis services are designed to respond to a crisis and offer treatment that is less restrictive and less stigmatising than hospitalisation. The development of a range of options, although slow, is happening where government has taken the lead. The present-day emphasis on a mixed economy of providers does not in itself produce variety. As smaller community-based units proliferate the danger is that what is created is simply smaller hospitals, which are of course less efficient than a larger hospital that is provided by a single provider. The government has increased the level of funding that is available to mental health services to help finance diverse provision.

If you had a blank sheet of paper and funding was assured, what alternatives to hospital would you wish to establish? How would you cater for minority mental health needs?

COMMENT

One of the key components in your deliberations about services ought to have been to work out with service users what they want or feel that they need.

Crisis services have become the new policy initiatives as they offer the potential of arresting a difficult situation before it becomes a full-blown emergency and escalates into a hospital admission. Your list could have included:

- *crisis intervention teams;*
- *24-hour crisis centres that can include short-term residential facilities;*
- *safe houses that offer less intensive experiences than the crisis centres;*

- *home treatment services where a multi-disciplinary team can support service users in their own homes;*
- *24-hour telephone support;*
- *specialist services for people from black and minority ethnic communities.*

What service users want in a crisis

Most of all what service users want is not to have any more psychiatric emergencies but if they do, they want a service that is responsive to their needs and provides a range of alternatives to hospital admission. Top of the service user list is a feeling of being in control of their own crisis. This included being involved in:

- crisis pre-planning;
- choice of treatments including complementary medicines;
- independent advocates; and
- access to quality information.

They also want to have someone to listen to them and to understand their explanation of what their crisis is about. Listening is an active process and social workers need to be skilled at this process and be prepared to spend time listening to them and not simply using the interview to detect signposts that assist with diagnosis (Golightley, 1985).

Some service users who have experienced a number of crises have developed their own checklist of what to do and what not to do when they are experiencing difficulty. This can include how to respond when they say that they do not want to take their medication when it is apparent that they are in distress. Another example is how to respond to them when they say that they are hearing voices. The point that they make is that making such a list is relatively easy when they are feeling well and upbeat but when they are distressed they recognise that they can lose their sense of what is best for them.

Intervention

The advent of the current legislations was thought to provide the means for an innovative service, which started from where the service user is rather than from what the available resources are. Thus the care co-ordinator should use his/her imagination to examine the best way of meeting the needs that have been identified in the assessment.

The most likely success will come from a treatment approach that will embrace a combination of anti-depressants and psychosocial support. The results of research suggest that this combination works and is more effective than either psychosocial intervention or medication on their own.[1] The psychosocial intervention could be a form of cognitive behaviour therapy; task-centred work or solution-focused work.

---

1 See Pritchard, 1995, p.122 for a detailed discussion of the combination of treatments.

This would be in addition to work with the more social aspects such as finances and isolation. With this in mind let us return to our case study and Mr Skeffling (Figure 6.1).

On this visual note the influencing factors have been noted. This could be taken further by the use of dotted lines where some aspects are weaker than others or by using as above different lengths of line and point. This gives a quick and easy picture of the challenges that are facing Mr Skeffling.

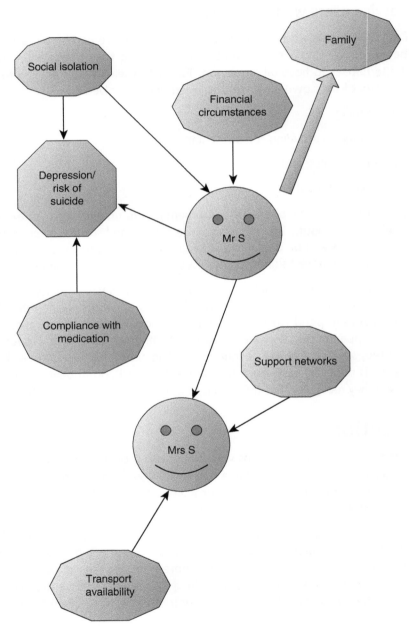

Figure 6.1   Visual representations of Mr Skeffling's psycho-social needs

> ## ACTIVITY 6.5
>
> *Using the visual note try to work out what the team could actually do to make Mr Skeffling feel more happy and more connected to his world. Take each oval and write down two or three tasks or aims. Once you have done this try to prioritise which ones should be tackled first and think about why this is so.*
>
> ### COMMENT
>
> *Taking your list you could now put them into categories such as those that stabilise the situation, those that will maintain him at home, those that support the clinical input, those that bring about personal growth and enhance coping skills and those that help to improve his social interaction with his wife.*

Needs or wants

One of the long running debates is the choice between what the service user may express as their want and what you and other professionals assess as their needs. Preferences may be expressed for example for a course of psychoanalysis by a service user but the cost of this is so prohibitive that it is seldom funded through the NHS. The allocation of scarce resources will always make some decisions difficult and make the realities of empowerment a challenge for social workers to meet.

Empowerment must remain the aim as well as equal opportunities and anti-oppressive practice. To practise in such a principled manner is also to work in what was called in Chapter 1 a culturally sensitive way. This is also necessary as all decisions are open to greater scrutiny since the enactment of the Human Rights Act 1998. Under s. 47(1) of the NHSCCA 1990 provision is made for the assessment of the need for community care services. This opens up the prospect of service users being unhappy with the assessment because it doesn't meet their wants as it is based on an assessment of a professional's view of their needs.

Mrs Skeffling can of course complain, as could Mr Skeffling. There is a precise complaints procedure that allows first the complaint to be resolved locally and then if that is not to her satisfaction it can move up the hierarchy. All local authorities and other care providers must show in writing how a complaint can be made. As a social worker you must inform service users and carers of their rights to complain (NHSCCA s.50). She is also entitled to her own assessment of her needs carried out in tandem with the assessment of her husband's (Johns, 2003).

CASE STUDY *continued*

Mrs Skeffling is unhappy with the services that have been provided for her husband.

You may want to consider the idea of 'spiritual healing', which has been developed by John Swinton (2001) in his interesting book *Spirituality and Mental Health Care*. Whatever your views might be about the place of spirituality, it is the case that for many users and carers spirituality is a very important concept. Swinton puts forward a model of social care that includes a spiritual dimension:

> *Care that takes seriously the spiritual dimensions of human beings requires an approach that draws carers into the deepest, most mysterious realms of human experience and allows them to function empathetically within a context that is often strange and alien.*

(Swinton, p.136)

The question which he rightly poses is how this approach can be made accessible to people who have mental health problems. The answer if indeed there is a single answer starts with focus being placed on the people themselves rather than on the implications of their diagnosis. This requires using a different approach and asking of the service user 'What gives the service user's life meaning?' And what can be done to enhance their meaning and connectedness?

Swinton suggests that such a basic refocusing enables the professional to see the situation as the service user sees it and to accept as valid the person's concerns rather than seeing the service user as a diagnostic entity. At its best this is a developed and deep communication with the service user. This is close to my ideas of phenomenology (Chapter 2, p. 55) which is a way of psychiatrists and others using empathy at the heart of their approach.

Swinton takes this on further by arguing that serious attempts to 'walk in the service user's shoes' mean that we need to learn a whole new language and ideas. The term 'interpathy' has been coined to describe the entry into the world of the service user and the genuine way of attempting to understand what he or she is experiencing. This is more than empathy as it has the extra dimension of exploration of the service user's world.

Social workers have an important part to play in this process as one of the few professionals who can interact with the service user, their families and community. The skills that you have learned and are learning should put you in a good position to be able to help others as well as yourself to understand service users and, if you choose to work in this way, to help them to find spiritual meaning in their lives.

Providing for individual need

By now you should be able to see that the most effective intervention will be based upon an accurate and negotiated assessment of needs that has been agreed between the service user and the professionals. The actual provision of services will vary depending upon the individual's circumstances and the imagination of the care co-ordinator and of course the assessment of eligibility.

ACTIVITY 6.6

Sketch out what your plan would be and check out the extent to which it meets the visual note.

My plan would be:

- *To provide individual work with Mr Skeffling. This could be in the form of cognitive therapy. The aim is to help him to increase his coping skills.*

- *To provide information for the family about the nature of depression and suicide.*

- *To ensure that he has a copy of the Charter, which gives him information about his rights, including the right to complain.*

- *To help him consider using direct payments to provide transport to the therapeutic day centre and to see the doctor. He would also like to attend a stress reduction class. To help him to enroll on the nearby history class which will also require daytime transport.*

- *To encourage him to go the CAB to have a financial makeover as there is a strong possibility that they are under-claiming benefits.*

- *To provide a short series of couple work to help them to look at their relationship and to respond to some of the anxieties and fears that Mrs Skeffling has which may be manifesting in her attitude towards him.*

- *To use the local MIND office to identify social support networks and to put him in touch with the local user group. They have older persons' groups and a day centre run by the members for the members. This will provide an easy route to helping Mr Skeffling to develop a network. Maintaining a network is much easier than starting one up from scratch.*

- *To arrange for a support worker to meet with him and go with him to the shops and get a coffee. This can also be used to encourage him to take his medication. This could be an effective use of direct payments. One of the aims is for him to develop a positive relationship whereby Mr Skeffling feels that he always has someone he can call if he needs to.*

- *To work with him to encourage and motivate him to want to get better and to do so by continuing to take his medication. As this has been a problem for him in the past this should be high priority.*

- *To work with Mr Skeffling to help him to write in a diary on a daily basis how he is feeling and what challenges he has faced. This will enable him to look back with his social worker to identify any patterns that might exist and to be able to recognise these and find ways of dealing with them.*

- *To develop with him a contract as the basis for future work. This will specify mutual expectations as well as what he wants people to do if it is noticed that he is becoming withdrawn or talking about it all being too much. This could also include keeping a diary record of his drinking habits.*

- *To arrange that he visits the 'crisis centre' and makes some contact with them. Now he is in the system he can access the services there should the need arise and there is a 24-hour help line. There is a short stay residential facility at the centre, which can be accessed through a professional referral.*

Monitoring and review

Like all plans they should be regarded as work in progress and subject to modification if and when the situation dictates. The best plans are those that all parties understand and of which they have shared ownership. Mr Skeffling at present is positive and wanting to develop his coping skills and to improve his relationship with his wife. The plan can facilitate this to happen but may need to be modified as people react differently to change.

CHAPTER SUMMARY

In this chapter you have explored working with service users who need services from time to time. The emerging forms of community care, if used imaginatively and with adequate funding, should offer service users improved services. Community care assessment is crucial to this process and in this chapter the example of an older man who is depressed and potentially suicidal has been used to illustrate some of the key points that social workers must understand in order that they can play a central role in the provision of community services.

Imagination and innovation are probably not the first words most people would use to describe the process of assessment and planning but they are essential attributes that need to be a part of the overall empowering approach. Situations like the case study are often complex and to work effectively you will need to understand not just your role but how that fits in with other professionals. You will find it difficult to be empowering of others when you are unsure yourself.

FURTHER READING

Wlliams, R. and Gethin Morgan, H. (eds) (1994) *Suicide Prevention: The challenge confronted: A manual of guidance for the purchasers and providers of mental health care.* NHS Health Service Thematic Reviews.

Well worth reading and contains useful checklists and discussion.

Colin Pritchard's book *Suicide – The Ultimate Rejection.*

Contains most of what you need to learn about the psycho-social aspects of working to predict and prevent suicide. It was published in 1995 and although parts are getting a little tired it is heading towards becoming a classic read.

WEBSITES

Useful organisations include:

Depression Alliance: **www.depressionalliance.org/**

MIND: **www.mind.org.uk/**

National Self-Harm Network: **www.nshn.co.uk/**

Survivors Speak Out: **www.gude-informatom.org.uk**

Values into Action: **www.viauk.org**

Mental Health Foundation: **www.mentalhealth.org.uk**

Management of depression in older people: **http://www.rcgp.org.uk/clinical-and-research/clinical-resources**

Chapter 7

Working with vulnerable people: adults who are long-term service users

This chapter will help you to develop the following capabilities from the **Professional Capabilities Framework:**

- **Professionalism**
  Identify and behave as a professional social worker committed to professional development.

- **Values and ethics**
  Apply social work ethical principles and values to guide professional practice.

- **Diversity**
  Recognise diversity and apply anti-discriminatory and anti-oppressive principles in practice.

- **Rights, justice and economic wellbeing**
  Advance human rights and promote social justice and economic wellbeing.

- **Knowledge**
  Apply knowledge of social sciences, law and social work practice theory.

- **Critical reflection and analysis**
  Apply critical reflection and analysis to inform and provide a rationale for professional decision-making.

- **Intervention and skills**
  Use judgement and authority to intervene with individuals, families and communities to promote independence, provide support and prevent harm, neglect and abuse.

- **Contexts and organisations.**
  Engage with, inform, and adapt to changing contexts that shape practice. Operate effectively within your own organisational frameworks and contribute to the development of services and organisations. Operate effectively within multi-agency and inter-professional settings.

It will also introduce you to the following standards as set out in the 2008 social work subject benchmark statement:

5.1.1   Social work services, service users and carers.
5.1.3   Values and ethics.
5.1.5   The nature of social work practice.

Introduction

This chapter will help you understand the type of social work to use when working with long-term and enduring mental health service users. The example of social work with people who have a diagnosis of schizophrenia is used to illustrate various aspects that are important when engaging with long-term service users. This will help you to understand the role that social workers and other professionals play in the treatment of people with schizophrenia. You will find it helpful to re-read Chapter 2 especially the Elyn Saks material. Working with long-term users can be a very demanding task and brings to the fore issues about liberty, dangerousness and the different parts that we all can play in the management of mental disorder.

> *It isn't that they can't see the solution. It is that they can't see the problem.*

G.K. Chesterton (1935)

Social work is an applied subject and:

> *… is characterised by a distinctive focus on practice in complex social situations to promote and protect individual and collective well-being. At honours degree level the study of social work involves the integrated study of subject specific knowledge, skills and values and the critical application of research knowledge from the social and human sciences (and closely related domains) to inform understanding and to underpin action, reflection and evaluation.*

(Subject benchmark statement 4.1.1)

Nowhere is this more relevant than in working with vulnerable people who have enduring or chronic forms of mental disorder, such as schizophrenia. This chapter will bring together some of the learning that has taken place in previous chapters about values and ethics, legal processes and context and understanding about mental disorder and some of the forms of treatment. Unlike the first four chapters in this book the last four start from the world of practice to give you the opportunity of learning about work with specific mental disorders.

Long-term users who experience schizophrenia

CASE STUDY

John is a mature student at university who lives with his father and his stepmother in an inner city area. He was admitted to the local psychiatric hospital on Saturday evening following an incident in which the police were involved. The events surrounding the admission are unclear, but it seems that John's stepmother had called the social services duty team when his behaviour became extreme and she felt threatened.

The next steps taken were to read John's file and to begin to refine an understanding of what had happened. The files make interesting reading and tell the story of a person who has been diagnosed as having paranoid schizophrenia and has been drifting in and out of contact with the services over the last five or so years. There is some evidence that he regularly abuses alcohol and that he likes to use recreational drugs such as cannabis and ecstasy. As a strong man he can present a rather threatening manner to people who annoy him and the previous social worker says that he has a 'short fuse'.

The visit to the home is quite illuminating as both John's father and his stepmother initially present themselves as well-educated, caring people. However as the interview progresses it becomes clear that while they may be caring, they are very critical of John and his social attitude and general behaviour. His father regards it as a failure that he is unable to live up to the brother's example. He went to Cambridge University, lives and works in London and is a bright person with a lot of friends. When his father divorced and remarried John's stepmother he thought that John had not got used to the idea of being in a new family and sometimes she felt his behaviour was simply to wreck her relationship with his father.

They both felt that John needed sorting out and that the services repeatedly let them down. They said that he was a danger to others when 'ill' and yet no one seemed to be interested in their view.

The initial contact

As a social worker you have picked up this case on Monday morning when you arrived at the office. There is a handwritten report from the duty Approved Mental Health Professional (AMHP) following John's admission to hospital. It appears that he was persuaded to go into hospital on an informal basis and is there now.

Multiethnic society

ACTIVITY 7.1

No mention has been made of whether John was from a minority ethnic group. What assumptions, if any, did you make about this? What difference would it make if John were African-Caribbean? Can you recall the impact of mental health in the black and minority ethnic communities?

COMMENT

Effective social work practice is one that is culturally sensitive, appropriate and examines personal, social and structural explanations for mental disorder. However to do this well you need to know about the different impacts that mental disorder has on people and, in the case of African-Caribbean young men, they are much more likely than their white majority equivalents to be admitted compulsorily under the MHA 1983. Figures do vary but one reliable and possibly conservative estimate is that African-Caribbean men are three times more likely to be admitted. Some medical practitioners suggest that stigmatisation and racism are likely to account for these differences in admission rates (Bhopal, 1998).

Assessment: the first stage

The gathering of information is an essential part of preparing for effective intervention (see Parker and Bradley, 2003). This process will probably be familiar to you and diagrammatically looks like this.

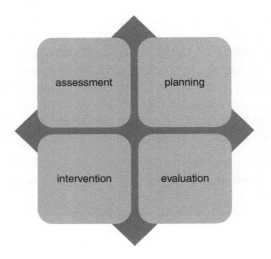

Figure 7.1

Assessment consists of a number of possibilities. In this case it could include:

- gathering information from the user's file which helps to paint a picture of the sort of contact that has gone on with this service user and under what circumstances;

- meeting with the stakeholders – a modernist term that includes the service user and his/her family or carer;

- discussion with the other professionals who are involved with the service user.

With this in mind the case file shows that similar incidents have occurred three times over the last couple of years and John has been detained on two of those occasions. He has been in and out of employment and decided this year that he would start at university with a view to a career in the health and social care professions. John has had several social workers including a student social worker over this period and the file has some major gaps. Unfortunately keeping accurate and up-to-date records is often treated as low priority by many social workers and it is at times like this that it becomes obvious that this means a certain degree of starting over again. When users have been detained in hospital there is a statutory requirement that a care plan should be completed and that this needs to involve the stakeholders who include John, his father and stepmother. When this has been properly carried out it will provide the full cycle of assessment, planning, intervention and evaluation for work with the service user up to the point that it is considered that the service user no longer requires this level of service.

The picture that is emerging is of a young man who has few friends and lives with his father and stepmother. He has few outside interests and the file shows that the relationships at home are not very supportive.

Dangerousness: who decides

Care in the community has had consistently bad press since the move to close down many hospitals and to relocate the service in the community. The killing in 1992 of Jonathan Zito by Christopher Clunis at a London underground station caught the public imagination and created a form of moral panic. The linking by the media, ever since Zito, of dangerousness and mental health has meant that the few incidents that have been reported have left an impression in the public mind that is difficult to erase. The effect of this has been unnecessary fear and also to put mental health professionals in the front line where any mistakes are very public.

The reality is that the thousands of decisions that are made correctly seldom get coverage. For those of you who are football fans the mental health professional is rather like the goalkeeper who makes hundreds of saves and is hardly noticed but if one error is made no one lets him/her forget. This is not to condone poor practice, as this needs eradicating where it exists, but in work that is necessarily complex and involves risk management things will not always work out as you predicted.

In spite of the above it is important that we study the cases where things have gone wrong and make sure that we learn from them. Subsequent inquiries have been well reported and in general show a degree of what is called 'system failure' characterised by a breakdown in communication and understanding between the various agencies that are involved. This has in turn resulted in a lack of trust not only by the public in services, but also it seems by government ministers who seem to be ever more influenced by interest groups as well as the impact of adverse publicity. However, this degree of panic reaction has and is being conducted largely in a research vacuum. The reality is that we simply do not know if the public is at an increased level of risk from mentally disordered patients (Coid, 1996).

CASE STUDY

When things go wrong!

In 2003, 19-year-old Daniel Rogerson was convicted of manslaughter with diminished responsibility after attacking and stabbing to death a 78-year-old neighbour in a sleepy village in Lancashire. In another instance Paul Kahn attacked and killed a complete stranger called Brian Dodd on a North Wales beach. Both of the attackers were people who were known to the services and had a history of severe mental illness. Both had a history of carers having sought help from services and in their opinions not receiving an adequate response.

However the evidence that is available shows that although the incidences are in reality very low, there are a small number of people who are likely to engage in violent acts. The latest conclusions in the *The National Confidential Inquiry into Suicide and Homicide by People with Mental Illness Annual Report* (July 2013, p. 51) are that 'the figures for homicide by patients with schizophrenia in 2009–2011 are the lowest in the report period and the lowest since data collection began in 1997'. It is evident that people with severe mental disorder who exhibit violent behaviour are much more likely to kill themselves rather than others.

The ability to predict who will carry out such acts is limited and far from a science. With this in mind Coid calls for:

- *better training for mental health professionals in assessment and treatment;*

- *more effective training in risk assessment and management; and*

- *patients who behave dangerously and default from treatment should not be allowed to become ill in the community.*

(Coid, p.967)

In John's case there was concern about his behaviour, but there was no evidence that he was actually violent. It is important to distinguish between what is verifiable evidence and what is speculation. Among the factors that need to be considered are:

- past history of violence which is the most reliable means of determining future conduct;

- poor compliance with treatment and aftercare;

- substance misuse; and

- recent severe stress.

This stage is still about gathering information about John and trying to determine what this episode means for him and his family. Once you have got about as much information as you are going to get, the next step is to determine what to do with the information.

Involving service users in risk assessment and management

Research commissioned by the Joseph Rowntree Foundation examined the involvement of users in their own risk assessment and management. The work was carried out in England and interviews were in-depth with users, carers and professionals. The findings include:

> *Many service users were aware that they could pose a risk to other people when experiencing psychosis and wanted to reduce the chances of this happening. Levels of agreement between service users and professionals about risk and how to respond to it ranged from full agreement to very little or none; and serious gaps were sometimes found in information held about service users that potentially put themselves and others at risk.*

(Joseph Rowntree Foundation, April 2004)

This shows that there is a lack of consistency in the overall approach to working with risk and risk management and much depends upon the individual professional. The researchers suggest that there needs to be a format for assessing risk and the subsequent management plan incorporates service users' views (Langan and Lindow, 2004).

The hospital visit

Shortly after the family has been interviewed John is visited on the ward. An initial and brief conversation with the nurse in charge reveals that John is in quite a distressed state and is receiving anti-psychotic medications. He is hearing voices and can exhibit challenging behaviour from time to time. The initial diagnosis has been confirmed as paranoid schizophrenia. This is also an important time for you to discuss with the nurse your safety when meeting with John. It is not the time for bravado as putting yourself in a potentially dangerous position is good for neither you nor John. In this instance the view is that the situation is safe, but as a precaution you are given a waist fitting alarm.

An investigation by the BBC News and *Community Care* magazine showed that in 53 Mental Health Trusts that 1,711 beds were closed since April 2011 representing a 9% reduction in the total number of beds that are available for people like John. One effect of this has been to place less seriously ill patients alongside extremely ill patients with very disturbed behaviour patterns. So much for psychiatric hospitals offering therapeutic respite. A national study conducted by Meehan and colleagues looked at suicide in patients admitted to psychiatric hospitals and revealed that a quarter of all inpatient suicides occurred within the first week of admission and on discharge the most frequent was in the first two weeks after leaving hospital, with the highest number occurring on the first day (*Br J Psychiatry*, 2013). Being admitted to a psychiatric ward is not always the best option for people and it is important to recognise that when this happens that everyone is alert to patients who may experience this as being very stressful and frightening, and discharge needs careful planning with community follow up and close supervision.

Understanding the impact of schizophrenia

In Chapter 2 some of the characteristics of schizophrenia were described which is information that you would need to know prior to your visit with John to enable you to discuss the treatment and care plan for John with the other professionals. The model that was used in this chapter suggests that even with disorders that have a physiological or genetic component to them, stress plays an important part. People with schizophrenia have a high sensitivity to stressful events, which can trigger the onset of an episode of schizophrenia. Such events can be located in life events such as divorce or loss of someone close to them, but could also include the loss of work or other events outside of their personal or family domain.

One of the features of some forms of schizophrenia is the experience of auditory hallucinations, commonly known as 'hearing voices'. Some people who have schizophrenia also have feelings of thoughts being inserted into their mind or have visual hallucinations. Interestingly these are usually culturally specific with people in the west hearing voices from space or computers while people from less developed countries may report hearing voices that are more to do with religion or demonic possession.

Understanding what the arrival of schizophrenia must mean to people is crucial for you as a social worker. We talk about walking in the other person's shoes and you should find whatever source you can in order to do this. You may be fortunate in that on your course there are service users who have had mental health experiences and they might be willing to share these experiences with you.

Understanding visual hallucinations is a feature of the movie A Beautiful Mind *that shows the life of the brilliant professor John Nash who works at an Ivy League university in the USA and has been a lifetime sufferer from schizophrenia that includes visual hallucinations. If possible try to see this film.*

Working with people who are hearing voices and experiencing delusions

Katie Glover (2000) has written a very practical guide for communicating with people who have mental health problems and there are some other guides that will help you to understand the best way of working with people who experience delusions or hallucinations.

There are some very practical steps including:

- *Recognition that the service user is experiencing voices instead of ignoring them and trying to carry on as if nothing was happening: 'Are you having difficulty following what I am saying?' 'Are you hearing voices?'*

- *Acknowledge the difficulty and distress that are caused by hearing voices: 'It must be very hard for you to continue with this conversation; thank you for sticking with it.'*

(Glover, 2000, p.157)

If John has said that it is very distressing you need to acknowledge that you understand and then be prepared to wait for a while or to postpone your interview. What you do not do is be dismissive of John's voices. They are real for him and you are starting from where he is.

Some people experience delusions which means that they are confused about who they are or often where they are. This can be disturbing for the family and disconcerting even for professionals. By and large the work that you would do with people who are deluded is simply a mixture of empathy and honesty. Consequently, faced with someone who says that they are from the secret service you might suggest, 'But now you are in this hospital and I want to work out with you how we can best help you.' This approach acknowledges the presence of the 'delusion' but avoids collusion with it and tries to establish a foothold in reality.

Hospitalisation

John is in hospital on an informal basis which means he can discharge himself at any time, subject to the holding power that is Section 5, MHA 1983, which gives nurses and doctors the right, in certain clearly defined circumstances, to keep John on the ward until a doctor can reassess his condition and evaluate the risks to John or to others (Chapter 3 covers this aspect). He is on an acute admission ward that specialises in the assessment of a patient's disorder and attempts to discharge as soon as possible. John is known to the services, consequently the assessment will not be to determine if he has schizophrenia, but to try to stabilise his current situation to the point where John can return home and a community treatment plan can be agreed between the stakeholders.

As we have seen in Chapter 3, informal patients can refuse treatment in line with common law. This right to refuse can be mediated if the patient is assessed as not having the capacity to make such decisions. Questions around capacity or lack of capacity are ones that medical practitioners have to address, often consulting with other professionals.

John is reasonably content to take his medication which the Responsible Clinician has prescribed and which includes anti-psychotic medication. This follows, you have learnt, a typical pattern for John. He will take his medication when in hospital and for a short while after discharge back to the community but he then stops his medication or becomes erratic in his self-administration. Changing this into a more reliable pattern becomes one of the goals for his treatment in the community.

If John had been detained on a section of the Mental Health Act 1983 the staff would be obliged to ensure that John was given specific information as soon as practicable about his admission and other information including rights about treatment, detention, renewal and discharge (s.132). This is considered to be good practice and similar information should be made available to John as an informal patient.

Life on the ward is a return to the familiar for John, but even so his experiences have not been overwhelmingly positive. This fits with evaluations of many service users who report concerns about:

- feelings of being unsafe on the ward;

- lack of meaningful activities to keep them occupied;

- insufficient information about their disorder and expectations of the ward staff;

- low levels of one-to-one interaction with the professional staff; and

- lack of involvement with planning their treatment and return to the community.

(See DoH, *Mental Health Implementation Guide*, 2002)

Many service users report the importance to them of one or two individuals with whom they had made a significant relationship or the importance of the other service users who helped them to get through the difficulties that they were in. But others feel that they were largely ignored and saw the RMO insufficiently for it to be a major factor in their recovery.

Substance abuse has also emerged as a problem on many acute admissions wards. Staff have to be vigilant to prevent the use of recreational drugs such as crack cocaine on the ward. This not only confuses the treatment regime of patients but can have an impact on the life of the ward in general and other patients in particular. Dual diagnosis is the term used to describe the coexistence of mental disorder with another diagnosis. This can be mental disorder and learning disability or mental disorder and substance abuse. In some inner city areas as many as three patients in ten have a dual diagnosis involving substance abuse with the consequence that they spend longer in hospital than do single diagnosis patients and are up to four times more likely to commit acts of violence than those with the single diagnosis of schizophrenia (*Rethink Sane*, Zito Trust, 2003).

These challenges pose real problems for hospital staff and striking the balance between the need for formal observation and vigilance against drug dealers can result in a mass of rules and procedures, the net effect of which can make living on a ward more like being in a custodial institution rather than a hospital. Service users need to be listened to and engaged wherever possible in the running of the ward and their care. As a social worker you can help this by checking with the service user that they have received information abut admission and discharge and that they are aware of some of the basics like menus, where phones are, wi-fi and access to legal help if needed.

Planning for successful intervention: working across agencies

The Care Programme Approach (CPA) has meant that the planning for John's discharge has already got underway and an initial plan has been developed in conjunction with John and using information from the family. This is put alongside the diagnosis, the previous notes and the views of the medical practitioner and the nursing team.

Working across agencies and between professionals from different disciplines has long presented a challenge for professionals who are trying to deliver a community-based service that is effective. The introduction by the government of the National Service Framework and the Care Programme Approach (CPA) in 1991 was just two of the features of the present-day mental health service. The CPA is focused to provide effort and resources on the more serious cases, which will include all of those patients who have been detained compulsorily. The CPA should produce a holistic service that is coordinated and uses a key worker or care coordinator system that takes the lead in all aspects of the involvement with the service user (more detail is provided in Chapter 3).

Most social workers will who work in the statutory sector will be based at community mental health teams (CMHT) and often these have morphed into assertive outreach, crisis resolution teams or home treatment teams.

> *Crisis Resolution Home Treatment teams are really beginning to prove their worth in the NHS. They are providing significant benefits and increased satisfaction for service users and reducing pressure on hospital beds.*

However, a lack of resources and a lack of multi-disciplinary support are limiting what these teams can do. And not all of those who would benefit from this service are being considered for it. These issues need to be addressed if the service is to improve.

(Sir John Bourn, Head of the National Audit Office, 7 December 2007)

However the jury is really out on the effectiveness of crisis resolution and home treatment teams as The Cochrane Study found very little evidence that they helped to avoid readmission to hospital. One of the key aspects of this is an assumed common vision of how the service might work. In one study all the professionals thought that they had clear objectives and a commitment to involving service users. Central to this is the attitude of the workers who are involved and the few evaluations of this tend to show that among nurses, social workers and support workers there is a shared view and a desire to change practices to be more user-focused (Carpenter et al., 2003). However, implementation of these modernised services across the country is patchy and research carried out by the NHS Executive and the Social Services Inspectorate in 1997 confirmed that a seamless service that was user-focused and not resource driven, was still an ideal in many parts of the country that was waiting to be implemented (Bartlett and Sandlands, 2003).

The introduction of the National Service Framework (NSFMH) in 1999 set out seven specific standards for providers of services to meet and these included a range of services from community outreach to secure hospitals. The standards apply across the board to both health and social service providers, and standards four and five refer explicitly to inter-agency work and the importance of multi-disciplinary assessment. There is also enabling legislation in the form of the Health Act 1999 that enables local authorities and health authorities to transfer funds to each other in order to promote a seamless service and to generally improve the quality of the service.

When teams come together this creates a common approach, but it would be a mistake to think that this means that everyone has an equal say. In particular, according to anecdotal evidence, doctors and psychiatrists are ostensibly happy to be a part of the multi-disciplinary team, but only when they retain, to use an American football analogy, the quarterback position (the star position). When this is put alongside research it shows, not surprisingly, the acquiescence of the service user to medical practitioners. Low (2004) writes that what is missing is the concept of active interest and involvement of lay people or, in our terms, service users. The effect of this is to create a new hierarchy in which the service user still remains at the bottom, the professionals, other than doctors, are in agreement with each other while doctors are still on top.

Service users at the centre?

It was the recognition that service users needed to be at the centre of reforms that led the government to embark on a comprehensive listening process to enable the service user voice to be heard. The listening exercise, 'Your health, your care, your say', allowed the public to speak directly to ministers, health professionals, and each other on how improvements could be made to their local services. Included in the 143,000 contributions were those of many mental health service users and carers. This exercise resulted in July 2005 in the publication of a new White Paper.

The White Paper: Our health, our care, our say: a new direction for community services

This Paper recognises how NHS and social care services work together and how these services could adapt to provide individuals with the health and social care services they need closer to their homes. The White Paper, *Our health, our care, our say: a new direction for community services*, aims to:

- *change the way these services are provided in communities and make them as flexible as possible;*

- *provide a more personal service that is tailored to the specific health or social care needs of individuals;*

- *give patients and service users more control over the treatment they receive;*

- *work with health and social care professionals and services to get the most appropriate treatment or care for their needs.*

> (DoH White Paper: *Our health, our care, our say: a new direction for community services*, January, 2006)

To achieve these aims will require that all agencies learn to work better together and that service users and carers will have more say in the type of service that they wish for and need. This will give greater emphasis to ideas of partnership – something that training and educational courses will need to remember. A random sample of 262 people with enduring mental health problems found that:

> *Frameworks which helped people to participate in their own care included common assessment protocols and the identification of a single key worker or care coordinator. Social work practitioners skilled in family work were identified as being particularly suited to this role...and people who use services responded more positively where there had been joint training of social workers and community psychiatric nurses towards a common goal of person-centred practice and a care management model based on strengths.*

> (SCIE Research briefing 26: Mental health and social work, July 2008)

As far as John is concerned you are lucky to be working for one of the community mental health teams, and it is in this context that you are trying to plan with John a course of treatment and care that will help him to stabilise while in the hospital and eventually to make the important move into the community. Assertive Outreach teams are something of a new invention and in reality it is too early to pass judgement about their effectiveness.

ACTIVITY 7.3

Think about the realities of working together in one multi-disciplinary team and the notion that service users and workers are in acquiescence to medical practitioners. Is this a good thing? To what extent do you think that this is inevitable? What impact will this have on you if you are to work in a multi-disciplinary team?

COMMENT

Even after recovery from an acute phase, most patients struggle to reintegrate into the community. In John's case, there were few community links prior to hospitalisation so the task of reintegration is even more difficult. Where home life is difficult the importance of work and outside activities increases and part of your task may be to identify what is available in the community. This could include sheltered workshops, day centres, and hostel or user groups. A good supportive environment is often to be found at voluntary organisations like MIND, the mental health charity, or other active mental health groups.

Had John been detained on a treatment order (s.37, s.3, etc.) there is a duty on primary care trusts or health authorities and social services departments to provide, in co-operation with the voluntary and independent sector, aftercare services until they are satisfied that the user no longer needs this service. This has caused some local problems as the duty is placed on the area, which the user goes to on discharge. This has resulted in some arguments between authorities as to who is responsible and a ruling from the High Court that it is the area from which the patient came when admitted that bears the financial responsibility, with the exception of people who are of no fixed abode (Bartlett and Sandland, 2003).

ACTIVITY 7.4

If John lived in your area what resources would be available for him? It would be helpful to you if you could spend a little time looking around at just what is available. If you have a local MIND shop they usually have a list of the resources that are in your area and sometimes community mental health teams have similar information.

Early intervention

The frequent contact with services interspersed with periods of low or no contact is some times also referred to as the 'revolving door' and presents a challenge to services. These patterns seem to be entrenched for John, which is unfortunate as research suggests that a key determinant in a person's career as a mental health patient is the speedy and effective response to the initial episode (Frangou and Bryne, 2000).

The first episode, like it was in John's case, happens usually in the late teenage years or early twenties and probably, as with John, the behaviour can go undetected for several months or even longer. This is largely because of the contextual factors that include:

- erratic behaviour that is also a characteristic of late teenage years;
- the known use of recreational drugs like cannabis which confuse the symptoms of psychosis;
- the first signs may be negative ones such as withdrawal, social isolation, and emotional flattening, none of which on their own may cause significant concern; and
- people who hear voices are often reluctant to tell people of this partly because they feel that people will think of them as being mad!

Trigger events

The model used in Chapter 2 helps to conceptualise about the onset and some of the factors that can result in mental disorder such as schizophrenia. Whether the occurrence of an episode is as a result of some event which effectively triggers this, or whether it is inside the person is unclear. However the likelihood is that it is as a result of key events that produce considerable stress for the user.

ACTIVITY *7.5*

With the above in mind can you speculate what the triggers might be in John's case? Think of those that might be personal for John and those that are more social.

COMMENT

Trigger events could be the result of some 'unresolved' issue for John, which has left him conflicted; this might be something hugely significant like emotional or other abuse while growing up. It could also be as a result of a stressful event that he has been unable to resolve, this could be starting at university and not being able to make social contacts, exacerbated by living at home. It might also be a combination of these.

Although the lifetime prevalence of schizophrenia is about 1%, which may seem low to you, the impact of schizophrenia brings with it huge social and personal costs. People who are diagnosed with this severe disorder literally join another tribe and can become isolated. The impact of the disability can be understood in the same way that Oliver (1996) writes about the social model of disability. The disorder itself can have a significant impact upon the person and their families but this is magnified by the association in the public's mind with dangerousness and the difficulties that the public has in dealing with unusual and unpredictable behaviour.

Consequently it really is in everyone's interest that early recognition and an appropriate response are made. The use of medication in the first episode is reported as being more likely to succeed as in the initial phase the user may be more responsive to treatment (Frangou and Bryne, 2000). This can take the edge off the psychotic symptoms and be an effective maintenance tool but on its own is probably insufficient.

The prognosis for people diagnosed with schizophrenia is that about 80% will recover but over 70% will have a second episode within a five to seven year period (Frangou and Bryne, 2000). This suggests that treatment should be considered longer term than the initial episode and that long-term courses of anti-psychotic medication may be advised. However, the most likely successful recovery or maintenance is to be found when the medication is a part of the overall treatment plan and a more holistic approach is used. This fits in with the model that was covered in Chapter 2 that brought together the different components that may impact on and lead to a mental disorder such as schizophrenia.

Although the dominant paradigm is medical, the evidence that supports the primacy of a uni-directional approach is hard to find. As a social worker you need to guard against this approach being the only one that you will work with as it brings with it some consequences for the service user and can make your role a secondary one. The advantages of using a more holistic assessment and modelling approach are that you can begin to understand why more African-Caribbean young men are diagnosed with schizophrenia than their equivalent white male counterparts. It also helps you to understand the role that families can play in the onset of schizophrenia and, importantly, in the treatment.

Intervention

It is generally considered that family circumstances are important determinants of future success or relapse with people who have schizophrenia. The research shows that relapse is more likely for users who have a diagnosis of schizophrenia if, after a period of hospitalisation, they return to a family that is overly critical or is emotionally over involved and controlling (Brown, in Butler and Pritchard, 1983, p.90). This resulted in the development of a concept called **expressed emotion** (EE), and the rather surprising finding that users may fare better in the community if they do not return to their families.

Pharoah et al. (2000) conducted an evaluation of the effectiveness of family interventions for people with schizophrenia in line with the drive towards increasing the evidence base for various interventions. This evaluation took Brown's work as the starting point for their evaluation and has produced strong evidence that confirmed their work. Even so the use of this approach in a practice setting is limited and it has, by and large, been left to one or two researchers to 'promote' this approach. The work of Leff, Kuipers and Lam (2002) is an example of this approach being slowly spread to other practitioners (nurses and social workers) through the Thorn Initiative. This was an extensive course in psycho-education approaches pioneered by the Maudsley NHS Trust and the University of Manchester.

EE is a clinical concept and the presence of high expressed emotion has a high predictive value. EE is actually a research technique and measures things like critical comments, hostility and over involvement that in turn produce emotions of various strengths. Experiencing high EE can cause considerable stress for some people and, it seems, especially for people with schizophrenia. Work with families involves trying to get families to move from expressing the negative side of emotions to developing techniques and mechanisms that demonstrate the positive aspect of emotion.

Measuring expressed emotion can be carried out using a standardised assessment schedule using the Camberwell Family Interview (CFI) that was developed in the 1960s. The user's family usually completes this and, because the person has been admitted to hospital, the completion of the schedule occurs soon thereafter. Interviews are usually taped and then subject to analysis or scoring over three dimensions, which are:

- **criticism,** which is measured by scoring the number of overtly critical and specific comments that have been made;

- **hostility**, which is scored when there is rejection of the patient as a person or a combination of general criticism and rejection;

- **over involvement**, which includes exaggerated emotional responses, usually self-sacrifice and overly devoted behaviour, over protection that is inappropriate to the patient's age, and difficulties in maintaining boundaries.

This requires practice and training as the tone and content of the interview are also taken as measures of the expressed emotion.

The treatment model as expressed by Leff et al. (2002) is underpinned by a view that can be summarised as follows:

- Schizophrenia has a biological basis but people who are diagnosed are particularly sensitive to stressful events, which make them vulnerable to relapse.

- Family members need to join in with therapeutic work, as they are both affected by the arrival of schizophrenia and may have contributed unwittingly to the relapse and possible onset.

- Honesty, openness and clear communication are important in order to share information about the nature of the disorder and to recognise the limitations of this knowledge.

- Families have positive as well as negative features and it is important to build on the strengths.

- This form of work needs to be carried out together with other forms of intervention and supervision.

As you can see, this is, in reality, a psychosocial education form of intervention in which your role as a social worker is to play the role of educator with the family. While social workers need to be aware of the medical side of mental disorder it is important that they retain their own skill base and capacity to work in an empowering way. This approach is empowering as the family is encouraged to learn more about schizophrenia and to work with the therapists to determine their own solutions to the problems as they see them.

Evidence is being gathered from other countries, which shows similar results to that achieved in the UK. Kalfi and Torabi (1996) carried out a study in Iran that included a cross-cultural comparison. This revealed that EE is an important factor in predicting relapse among users who have schizophrenia who lived in Iran. In a similar vein studies about the impact of high EE in families that contain a user with bipolar disorder or unipolar disorder also look promising.

While to become fully competent in this type of intervention does require additional training, the general principles of these approaches can be usefully applied to many situations. As a social worker you could be the champion of an approach that is empowering of the service user while retaining the treatment ethos of a uni-directional approach. This approach encapsulates social factors such as unemployment, substance misuse, poor social networks, and high expressed emotions and puts them alongside the diagnosis of mental disorder as equal partners rather than as subsidiary parts (Tew, 2002).

Working with John and his parents in a holistic manner puts them centre stage and offers them the opportunity to learn about schizophrenia and to understand the effect that their communication patterns may have upon John. In some cases it may be advisable for John to leave his parents' home and to live in other accommodation and 'manage' his relationship with his parents in this way. This enables him to escape the 'trapping' patterns of communication but also does not place the blame for his disorder on the parents. After all, it is very unlikely that parents consciously choose to relate to their children in ways that create problems.

Caring for the carers

Carers of people with long-term mental health use may find the process challenging and debilitating. Those carers who provide regular and substantial care for a person on CPA are covered by Standard Six of the National Service Framework, which to be met, would mean that they receive their own written care plan following discussions with them and your assessment of their physical and mental health needs. This needs to be carried out annually at least.

Assertive Outreach/home treatment

Assertive Outreach teams are a part of the reform to mental health services in the community. They work in an intensive manner with long-term users of mental health services who are considered to be difficult to engage in treatment. John would probably fall into this category given his history of non-compliance with medication and his readmissions to hospital.

The Sainsbury Centre, in 2003, reviewed the people skills that are needed to work with the typical service user who receives Assertive Outreach. They came up with a list of personal and professional attributes that included being able to:

- work with service users in informal settings;
- work with service users and families in an accepting and certainly uncritical manner;

- hold realistic expectations of service users and the scope for complete recovery; and

- relate to service users' experiences of mental health, possibly through their own experience of oppression or of mental health.

(Sainsbury Centre, 1998)

The same document also describes some of the evidence that underpins the assertive outreach approach and claims that they can reach a large percentage of hard-to-engage service users and that they are generally liked by service users and their carers. When these teams work well they provide an integrated service that consists of a variety of professional groups including community psychiatric nurses and social workers. Yet the impact of funding cuts is a major threat to some specialist services and in some cases has resulted in the merging of specialist crisis resolution and assertive outreach teams with the generic community mental health teams. The most recent report of the National Confidential Inquiry reported that 'since 2006 there have been more patient suicides under CR/HT than in in-patient care, reflecting a change in the nature of acute care. In the last 3 years over twice as many suicides have occurred under CR/HT'. This is turn prompted a recommendation to 'improve safety in crisis resolution/home treatment (CR/HT) as a priority for suicide prevention in mental health care; particular caution is needed with patients who live alone or refuse treatment and when patients are discharged from hospital into CR/HT' (2013, p.7).

ACTIVITY 7.6

Make some enquiries, if you do not already know, whether there is an Assertive Outreach team in the area in which you live. If they do exist, get their information for service users, which should help you to understand more about this specialised multi-disciplinary service.

Recovery

It is important to appreciate that it is not possible, perhaps not even desirable, to be able to 'cure' mental health problems. Sometimes the side effects of treatment are such that service users prefer to learn ways of coping with the symptoms of their illness. In January 2010 government policy appeared to support ideas of recovery (New Horizons, 2010) and described recovery as 'a way of living a satisfying, hopeful and contributing life, even with the limitations caused by illness. Recovery involves the development of new meaning and purpose in one's life as one grows beyond the catastrophic effects of mental illness' (Shepherd et al., 2008). The principles and practice involved are a good fit with social work practice; promoting hope, control, finding meaning, encouraging active participation and valuing relationships. However as Nathan and Webber point out social workers need to do their upmost to ensure that the underlying philosophy behind recovery informs the interventions and approach and that it doesn't become another word for 'rehabilitation' (Nathan and Webber, 2010, p.238).

A powerful account from a service user's perspective (much along the same lines as Saks in Chapter 1) is the article written by Patricia Deegan (1996) describing how she coped with recovery and describing the sort of services that we need to offer to help service users recover from mental health disorder. Her writing is powerful as witnessed by this except.

> *The concept of recovery is rooted in the simple but profound realization (sic) that people who have been diagnosed with mental illness are human beings. Like a pebble tossed into the center of a still pool, this fact radiates in ever larger ripples until every corner of academic and clinical practice are affected. Those of us who have been diagnosed are not objects to be acted on. We are fully human beings and we can speak for ourselves...*

and goes on to say

> *We can become experts in our own journey of recovery.*

(Deegan, 1996, p.92)

As she writes recovery of course does not mean cure and the journey will have gains and setbacks but service users need to be able to embark on this journey and be supported.

The plan

Your own understanding of the challenges that John faces and your assessment of the trigger events will inform your work with him. This is nearly always achieving a balance between what the service user wants, what you and other professionals think that the service user needs and the reality of what is actually available. The process should begin early and have the service user at the front of the deliberations about treatment options. The CPA assumes that the care plan will be drawn tighter with the active involvement of the service user and that they will have agreed and signed the action plan.

ACTIVITY 7.7

With John the plan could take on a number of different shapes and at this point with the little information that you have you should make some notes of three possible plans.

COMMENT

Your three plans would of course be drawn up following discussion with other professionals, John and his family. They might include (but not be limited to) these.

Plan one

Do nothing and let John leave hospital and return home taking anti-psychotic medication. They have your telephone number and if the situation worsens they can contact you. The

(Continued)

(Continued)

justification for this is that it's the least invasive plan and of course uses the least direct resources. This assumes that you have all decided that John is not a risk to either himself or to others.

Plan two

John returns home taking anti-psychotic medication, and with the offer of family work to reduce the level of expressed emotion in the family and with your support he will eventually return to university.

Plan three

John moves to supported living accommodation in town, his family are offered ten sessions to help them to understand how they can change some of their behaviours to help his recovery, he starts going to the local MIND day centre and takes part in a support group run by service users for people hearing voices. The local assertive outreach team offers him a package of comprehensive services including monitoring his medication.

CHAPTER SUMMARY

Several themes should be evident in this chapter, not least of which is working in partnership with service users. Because of the debilitating nature of schizophrenia and the low level of public knowledge about the condition you will have to move at a slow pace and be acting as both a therapist and a psycho-social educator. The use of a holistic assessment and psycho-social methods of working is likely to be the most effective social work intervention with people who have long-term schizophrenia (like John).

As a social worker you have a crucial role to play in holistic assessment and, in order to fulfil this role, you need to be a professionally competent worker who has sufficient knowledge to be able to hold your own with medical practitioners without unnecessary acquiescence to them. Your work should be characterised by empowerment, emotional engagement and networking including a high level of specific knowledge about the resources that you have available in your area and about what works.

FURTHER READING

Priebe, S. and Slade, M. (2002) *Evidence in Mental Health Care*. Hove: Brunner-Routledge.

Has some very useful chapters about what works and with whom. See the chapter on the user perspective about what counts as evidence.

For help and advice about benefits consult *The Big Book of Benefits and Mental Health*.

Neath Mind, 32 Victoria Gardens, Neath, SA11 3BH. A ten-page proforma is available online from **www. rightsnet.orguk/pdfs/AA**

Chapter 7Working with vulnerable people: adults who are long-term service users

National Audit Office (December 2007) *Helping People through Mental Health Crisis: The role of Crisis Resolution and Home Treatment services.*

University of Manchester (2013) National Confidential Inquiry into homicide and Suicide Annual report by people with mental illness – can be accessed at **www.bbmh.manchester.ac.uk/cmhr/ centreforsuicideprevention/nci/reports/NCIAnnualReport2013V2.pdf**

Huffington Post accessed 18/10/2013 at **www.huffingtonpost.co.uk/dr-raj.../nhs-complaints_b_ 4108370.html**

WEBSITES

Subject benchmark statements are best accessed through the Quality Assurance Agency (QAA) website: **www.QAA.ac.uk** and then into subject benchmarks.

Joseph Rowntree Foundation, York: **www.jrf.org.uk**

Chapter 8

Working across organisational and professional boundaries

Introduction

> *Sunlight is the most powerful of disinfectants and electric light the best policeman.*

Mr Justice Brandis (1914)

This final chapter brings together some of the themes from earlier chapters under the heading of working together to provide an integrated service that is efficient and effective. Providing an integrated service that will protect children is used as an example although the need to work together applies across the whole range of services. The links with other chapters, such as Chapter 5 on working with children and adolescents, will be all too apparent but in this chapter the primary focus is upon providing the service user with a needs-led service that does not involve them having to be referred to other agencies.

Children are rightly the focus of this chapter because they may be in need of mental health services because of individual mental disorder; they may be being parented by someone who is themselves experiencing mental disorder or they could be the unfortunate subject of a fabricated mental disorder. In the UK 2–5% of children are brought by their carers to the attention of Primary Care Teams with mental health issues as the main presenting problem. It is likely that many more children with mental health problems do not present at all (Spender et al., 2001).

At the extreme end the pressing issue of child protection and mental health is explored using the Victoria Climbié Inquiry (she died in 2000) and the death of Peter Connelly (Baby P) in 2007 as examples of the need to put children first, irrespective of different professional boundaries. This signalled a new approach brought in under the Labour government that may have started out as a straightforward response to the death of Victoria Climbié but soon became much more ambitious to try and ensure that children should have the chance to fulfil their potential and the introduction of Every Child Matters (ECM) that set out the five key outcomes for children to be 'healthy, stay safe, enjoy and achieve, make a positive contribution and experience economic well–being' (2003). This also resulted in reorganisation of services and the move from a reactive approach to an intervention where multi-professional concerns about the welfare of children were brought together through Sure Start Centres that in many cases have turned into Children's Centres.

With the change of government in 2010 came the name change for the Department of Children, Schools and Families, which reverted to the more traditional Department for Education and when Michael Gove took office it was as the Secretary of State for Education not children. This was of course when austerity was beginning to bite and among a raft of changes since the election of the coalition government was the not too subtle move from the 'five outcomes' of ECM to helping 'children to achieve'. There was no public disagreement with the overall concept of ECM, after all, who could disagree, but the new focus was to raise standards and performance of schools.

Community-based services have now become one of the dominant organisational forms from which mental health services are provided and this chapter will help students to understand the roles that they can perform in such services. These will include working as a 'care coordinator' to provide direct services and as an 'assessment officer' to determine the extent that services should and can be provided.

It is significant that in the very locality where Climbié and Connelly died there has been a transformation of services under a project called *Reclaiming Social Work*. The change agenda has created an environment where social work is finding its feet and looking towards 'evidence-based' interventions to help families to change their behaviours. Webber writes:

> *Clinicians are funded by local child and Adolescent Mental Health Services. Clinicians are embedded within units to undertake interventions, and to advise colleagues – hardwiring clinical thinking and clinical evidence within the units.*
>
> (Webber, 2010, p. 215)

Working with service users as individuals and with service user action groups has become a standard way of working but one that requires considerable skill and understanding, both of which are explored as an aid to student learning.

Major changes in 2013

Change is an ever-present feature of the world of mental health and many of the changes just coming in are as a result of the Heath and Social Care Act 2012. But these are structural changes and the actors are pretty much as they were before these changes occurred. Some of the changes reflect the policy of deciding services at a local level and also the present neo-liberal approach to the larger provision of services.

Healthwatch England was launched at a conference hosted by the Care Quality Commission (CQC) in October 2012 and set up a network of local healthwatch organisations that will represent the views of patients and the public. You may want to check out on the internet what your local Healthwatch is up to and there are also opportunities for you to get involved with them. They are set up to be an independent body with the following powers under the Health and Social Care Act 2012:

- To gather people's views on, and experiences of, the health and social care system.

- To send trained representatives to enter and view local services to speak to patients and service users, and observe services being delivered.

- To make reports and recommendations and to get a response from commissioners and service providers.

- To have influence on local commissioning decisions through membership of the statutory health and wellbeing board, and involvement in preparing joint health and wellbeing strategies.

And to alert Healthwatch England, or the CQC, where appropriate, to concerns about specific care providers, health or social care matters

From April 2012 GP **Clinical Commissioning Groups** (CCGs) took over the responsibility for the provision of mental health services in each locality. These groups must, by law, involve service users and have a duty to appoint lay members to the Board managing the CCG. At a national level a **NHS Commissioning Board** (NHS CB) is now operational to assess the quality of the CCGs as well as commissioning services that meet national need such as secure hospitals and police custody suites.

Health and Wellbeing Boards are also being set up in each area addressing present and future need for health and social care settings. They will carry out assessments called **Joint Strategic Needs Assessments** (JSNAs).

These groups are in place by law and they are decision-making bodies but, as alluded to in Chapter 1, though how they go about their work is for them to decide and it would be pointless to set up local bodies if all they did was to have the same priority as other services. They are new and looking for people to get involved, why not volunteer?

Service users' views

A development of these ideas is termed 'The Circle of Involvement', which is a simple way of understanding how it is necessary and what steps need to be taken to ensure that service users become more involved. This was conceived out of work that was carried out in the Trent region and brings together key components such as education and training, government policies, service development and workforce development. By visualising these components as a circle that is seamless and that one component feeds in to the other it is possible to work towards greater involvement at any stage (*Principles for Practice*, December 2005).

Involving service users owes its origins to the Children Act (1989 revised 2004) and the 1990 NHS and Community Care Act, both of which placed the involvement of service users on the agenda. The idea of citizen participation goes back much further than this and can be traced to town planning and the work of Sheri Arnstein (1969) who first developed a 'ladder of participation' and subsequently to the community social work and community development movements of the 1970s. This has gained considerable momentum with the requirement put onto social work courses to involve service users in all aspects of social work training. Where this is taken seriously it will undoubtedly be a transformatory process and could result in major changes to education and training. However, it is still too early to evaluate if the involvement of service users will be more than just a fine idea.

The mental health service user movement includes those that are involved at the governmental level such as MIND and YoungMinds, both of which regularly submit high quality detailed analyses to inform policymaking. There are few examples of patient controlled services but one is Camden Mind that has a track record of over 23 years of successfully delivering community mental health services. In addition there are local user groups, which may be affiliated to the national bodies such as SANE or MIND or Survivors Speak Out and specialist groups such as Women in Special Hospitals.

Service users need to be consulted about the services that they receive to help find out what sort of intervention works well and why. However, in contrast with clinical drugs trials, all too often the evaluations that have been carried out are about satisfaction with the services received when what is desperately needed is an evaluation of what worked and the extent to which it worked.

Service users can be involved at different levels:

- individual level where they work with the professionals to determine what is the most appropriate way of responding to their mental health needs;
- group level with service users working together, with or without professional facilitation, to support each other;

- activist groups where they comment upon aspects of service delivery and challenge or inform conventional operational practices;

- involvement at a strategic level to plan services or training courses such as service user groups or as individual representatives;

- involvement in national bodies to campaign for changes and to offer government policy-makers advice and assistance.

The involvement of service users varies according to what level they want to become involved at and what is available. At each level there is also the prospect that within that level will be specialist interests such as black and minority ethnic or women's groups. The key for social workers is to form alliances with service user groups and to work with them in ways that will recognise the contribution that both can make in moving towards a mental health service that is user-focused and emancipatory.

ACTIVITY **8.1**

Some organisations work as pressure groups campaigning for what they see as necessary changes to mental health law and services. Now is the time for you to go onto the internet and check out at least one of these sites. The YoungMinds website www.youngminds.org. uk is usually one of the best for a wide range of coverage of mental health issues.

COMMENT

The involvement of adult service users has been slow to get underway and at times appears somewhat tokenistic. However there has been even less progress with children and adolescent involvement. It is surprising given the legislation about children's rights that they can be so easily overlooked and the adult view of what children want dominates. Even the present proposals to reform the legislation state that when considering individual treatment for children and young people the clinical team must consider the wishes and feelings of the child while they must take 'proper account' of the parental view. This took into account the view that children may not be competent to determine their own treatment but this is seemingly contradictory with the Richardson Committee suggestion that children should be considered competent from the age of 10–12 and that competence should be assessed according to the Gillick judgement.

ACTIVITY **8.2**

What reasons can you come up with to explain why the perspectives of children and young people have not been considered in respect of mental health services? How valid is this? Would lowering the age at which people can vote to 16 make any difference?

The Equality Act 2010

The Equality Act came into force in October 2010 and brought together several previously separate acts. This has simplified the law in this area and also made it stronger in several areas. This has provided more impetus to involving people with mental health problems not only in their own care but in their involvement with services.

The Act sets out what is termed *protected characteristics,* which include age, disability (which includes mental health and people diagnosed as clinically obese), race, religion or belief, sex, sexual orientation, gender reassignment (people who are having or who have had a sex change, transvestites and transgender people), marriage and civil partnership, *and* pregnancy and maternity.

This will provide a certain degree of protection for people who are 'discriminated against by virtue of their disability' and importantly the legal definition of disability has been widened to include for example long-term depression where it significantly interferes with a person's day-to-day activities. For example, it will help protect employees suffering from depression from being unfairly discriminated against. It is also something that social work courses have to consider when making judgements about the suitability of students.

Under the Equality Act 2010 a **public sector Equality Duty** came into force across Great Britain on 5 April 2011: all public bodies have to consider all individuals when carrying out their day-to-day work – in shaping policy, in delivering services and in relation to their own employees. They must have due regard to:

(a) *eliminate discrimination, harassment, victimisation and any other conduct that is prohibited by or under this Act;*

(b) *advance equality of opportunity between persons who share a relevant protected characteristic and persons who do not share it;*

(c) *foster good relations between persons who share a relevant protected characteristic and persons who do not share it.*

(Equality Act 2010, s149.1)

Working towards an integrated service

The idea of working together to provide seamless service-to-service users is far from new. In 1976 as a part of a research team we published my first major piece of mental health research (Jones et al., 1985). This was a project led by Professor Kathleen Jones of York University and was a tracer study to examine the destinations of nearly 200 patients who had been discharged from York psychiatric hospitals over a two-year period. In that research we examined the ways that agencies tried to work together or to be more frank the ways that they didn't manage to work together! Back then we talked about agencies 'collaborating', a rather strange term given that collaboration means working with the enemy! Since then I have followed with personal and professional interest how things have moved on and it is timely to revisit the idea about working together.

Integrated services are services that are joined together to provide one access route for service users. Such services imply common training to at least some extent and shared values. Multi-disciplinary approaches retain the professional and often organisational identity of the professional involved.

Multi-disciplinary teams

The multi-disciplinary team exists both as a community mental health team, and in a form that includes professionals who work in the team part-time and also work back in their own agencies. A child mental health team could comprise members as in Figure 8.1, although this will vary from agency to agency. The first point for involvement will usually be a referral from the family doctor to this team for assessment and, if intervention is planned, a care coordinator will be appointed who will carry the responsibility for the case. This can be the scene for some power struggles between the professions and also within the professions. General practitioners are often more comfortable dealing with another medical colleague rather than relating to a professional from a different discipline. Consultants will point out that they have clinical responsibility for the individual and hence medical–legal responsibility. This

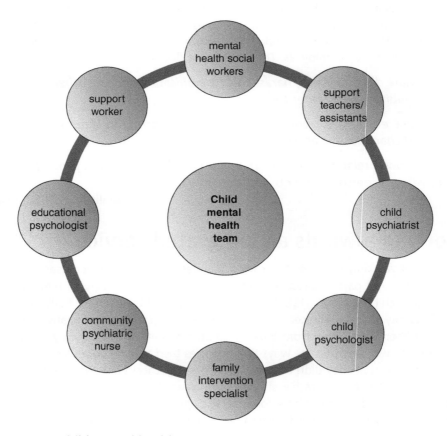

Figure 8.1   Child mental health team

has been further compounded with the emergence of nurse prescribers. These issues can be sorted out and it is important that the multi-disciplinary team establishes clear operating procedures. The core principle should be shared commitment to improve the lives of children and young people as enshrined in the Children Act 2004 section 10 a 'duty to co-operate'. The shift is towards doing this at a local level and this increased local autonomy is to be helped, in theory at least, by reductions in unnecessary bureaucracy and regulation.

The emergence of a new, planned workforce

The National Workforce Action Team was established to determine what the demand for staff might be and what type of staff was needed for the modernised mental health service. Poor workforce planning has resulted in much of the present services developing in an *ad hoc* way that reflects more circumstance, history and influence than effective planning. The slowness of establishing joint planning teams has hindered the development of widespread effective integrated services. The Workforce Action Team pointed out that poor planning was in part the result of the limited links that agencies had with each other and the general lack of enthusiasm across professions to implement flexible working practices and cooperation (Alcock, 2003).

One of the exciting developments in community mental health has been to recognise the importance of factors such as community support and networking. This is important work, which can make a huge difference to the experience of the service user. This has coincided with the emergence of a new support worker with a new type of qualification. These roles are close to those of social work but are more limited in their scope. Some professionals see this new form of worker as a threat to their role and simply a means by which government can cut the wage bill. What do you think?

The management of mental health professionals

Careful risk assessment is necessary for any person who is engaged in direct work with people who are under the age of 18 years and are provided with health or social care services, especially in the light of the Allitt Inquiry (see later in this chapter). This includes health screening to ensure that they are fit for employment and that any condition, which is revealed, can be managed in a way that will not adversely affect their work with service users or colleagues. This is a balancing act that requires careful assessment, especially in the light of the need to reduce discrimination that people with disabilities, including mental disorder, experience.

The list of Inquiries that permeate social work makes monumental reading but there are valuable lessons that must be learnt if the profession is to progress and vulnerable people be better served. It is to these that we briefly turn.

Learning from Inquiries

Two Inquiries are described, one concerning the circumstances around the death of Victoria Climbié and the other that of the nurse Beverley Allitt who was convicted of the murder of several children at the hospital ward where she worked. They are but two of many, far too many, Inquiries into the untimely death of people who in different ways had expected the services to have done more to protect them. Although each Inquiry has some specific lessons that need to be learned, together they point out that some of the basics that make up competent practice have not been taken on board.

The Victoria Climbié case

Victoria was a healthy, lively, happy young girl who had been sent to England by her mother in the hope that she would be well educated and achieve her potential. What parent would not want this for their child? However this was not to be and in the space of a few months she was tortured, humiliated and in the end died. At the post-mortem examination she had over 128 separate injuries all over her body. In the final few weeks of her life social workers made attempts to see Victoria but made the incorrect assumption that she and her carer had moved. That the result was tragic is self-evident but that it could have been prevented is a shocking indictment of professional services including social workers (Johns, 2003).

Were Victoria's carers mentally disordered or just sadistic people? There certainly is an argument that can be made to support the view that anyone who tortures and kills a person must be mentally disordered even though in this case the sentencing suggests that this was not an argument that found favour with the jury.

What lessons can be learned?

1. Social workers and other professionals should learn to listen to children and not to dismiss what they say. This needs to be put alongside observations that add to the child's explanation.

2. Social workers should be clear about the purpose of contact with service users and what information needs to be gathered to clarify levels of accountability (recommendation 5, Climbié).

3. Staffing levels, training and management are all in need of improvement and monitoring.

4. As far as mental health services are concerned the following has emerged:

   • more support for young carers is needed;

   • the overall approach should be multi-disciplinary with a lead professional involved; and

   • there should be a common assessment framework.

The Child and Adolescent Services (CAMHS) received additional funding to develop a more comprehensive approach to child mental health problems (see Chapter 5). In addition to these measures the various bodies charged with monitoring compliance with national standards are asking social services and trusts to provide information about the arrangements for safeguarding children and to ensure that their staff are suitably trained and aware of their responsibilities towards children.

This was not without irony or controversy as following Climbié schools were now tasked with looking after all aspects of pupils' lives and to do this a variety of measures emerged with breakfast clubs in most schools, closer links between police and Social Services. This was a huge investment of time and other resources but all for the undeniably good cause of safeguarding and protection of vulnerable children. But we all knew that such instances, though rare, cannot be totally prevented and Peter Connelly's death in 2007 showed that all the action that had occurred in the seven years between these events were insufficient to prevent horrific abuse finding its way through the cracks. The irony was that Every Child Matters, the flagship of the Labour government's response to Climbié was now blamed for Peter Connelly's death and change was afoot.

As Martin Shaw, editor of the *Times Educational Supplement* wrote, 'how had a former education director with a background as a head teacher ended up the boss of social workers? Why had Harringey's child protection work been inspected and given thumbs up by a schools watchdog? The answer was Every Child Matters' (**http:// emotionsblog.history.amul.ac.uk/?p=1378** accessed 28 November 2013).

BEST PRACTICE

Example of evidence-based parenting

The city of Salford has established a number of evidence-based parenting programmes – Baby Incredible Years, Incredible Years and Triple P – delivered across the city. These are based on existing research and are themselves evaluated programmes. They claim that evidence shows parents who participate become more competent and comfortable in their parenting role, have strengthened relationships with their children, and their overall family wellbeing increases. Parents develop skills to enhance their child's social, emotional and academic competency, and learn strategies to deal with difficult and challenging behaviour in consistent, non-punitive ways.

The target groups include:

- *parents whose children are subject to interim care orders (ICO), child protection plans, or children in need plans;*

- *parents whose children are at risk of offending;*

- *parents whose children display conduct disorders or have a diagnosis that affects their behaviour;*

- *parents who are finding it difficult to manage their child's behaviour and need a targeted group intervention.*

www.salford.gov.uk/parenting-programmes.htm *accessed 5 December 2013*

The Allitt Inquiry

In the early part of 1991 three children died suddenly and unexpectedly on the children's ward at Grantham and Kesteven General Hospital. There were further 'emergencies' later that year which finally aroused suspicion and a police investigation started. The suspicion was that someone was deliberately harming children on the ward. Eventually this was traced to a young nurse called Beverley Allitt who was subsequently charged with four murders, nine attempted murders and nine accounts of causing grievous bodily harm. While on duty in the children's ward in her local hospital, she tried to kill at least 23 children by injecting them with insulin and potassium, choking, breaking ribs and asphyxiation.

Beverley Allitt suffered from the rare Munchausen's Syndrome by Proxy (MSBP) which is a variation of Munchausen's Syndrome, in which individuals fake symptoms or harm themselves so that they can be the centre of attention. The syndrome is named after a German soldier renowned for telling exaggerated stories. There is still no convincing theory about the causes of this disorder and it is quite rare. Beverly Allitt was sentenced to 13 life sentences and was transferred to a high security psychiatric unit.

Sir Cecil Clothier conducted the Inquiry that followed in 1994. Among many findings was the following comment:

> *Taken in isolation, these fragments of medical evidence were not all very significant nor were the failure to recognise some of them very culpable. But collectively they would have amounted to an unmistakable portrait of malevolence. The principal failure of those concerned lay in not collecting together those pieces of evidence.*

> (Clothier, 1994, p.131)

There are concerns that over-vigilance may result in spurious identification of false risk, a topic that resulted in widespread discussion, including in the House of Lords where the possibility of such a condition being widespread was considered and the possibility of false diagnosis discussed (Lords Hansard, 1997).

> *Put at its simplest, there is all the difference in the world between a Beverley Allitt, whose severe personality disorder led her to murder young children, and a mother who invents reasons why she and her child should visit the doctor. Yet under the all-embracing banner of MSBP, and in the hands of the untrained, the two are treated as being practically indistinguishable. It does not matter whether one calls the condition MSBP or factitious illness by proxy, or by any other name. The point remains the same.*

> (Lords Hansard, 1997)

What lessons can be learned?

The Allitt Inquiry demonstrated four aspects that are particularly relevant for this chapter:

1. The need to look out for patterns that help to explain what otherwise might look to be phenomena that are unconnected. This means keeping an open mind and discussing your ideas with others.

2. The need to establish and operate a strong whistleblowing protocol that allows other professionals to raise concerns about questionable practice and for these to be followed up.

3. The importance of staff screening, and regular supervision and monitoring of performance.

4. The professional culture should be underpinned by values and driven by the empowering practice that is open to challenge.

In light of these Inquiries we need to ask ourselves just how we protect children who are at risk and promote their positive mental health and ability to cope with adverse and stressful situations.

Working together to safeguard children
The policy and legal context

The main legislation is the Children Act 1989, which applies to a person under the age of 18, and the Mental Health Act 1983. In March 2013 the statutory guidance was issued 'Working Together to Safeguard Children: A guide to inter-agency working to safeguard and promote the welfare of children'. (This document is available online at **www.education.gov.uk/aboutdfe/statutory** Reference: DFE-00030-2013) and it provides an easy-to-follow guidance.

What is the diference between safeguarding and child protection?

The Department for Education provides a useful answer to this question and defines safeguarding and protection as:

- protecting children from maltreatment;

- preventing impairment of children's health or development;

- ensuring children are growing up in circumstances consistent with the provision of safe and effective care;

- taking action to enable all children to have the best outcomes.

Child protection is a part of safeguarding and promoting welfare. It refers to the activity that is undertaken to protect specific children who are suffering, or likely to suffer, significant harm. (**www.education.gov.uk/popularquestios/a0064461/safe-guarding-and-child-protection** accessed 3 December 2013)

Various provisions in the Children Act (1989) permit the psychiatric examination of a child although once the child is of sufficient understanding, using the Gillick rules, the child can refuse to be examined (Eldergill, 1997). If the court decides that there is a chance of significant harm a Child Assessment Order (s.43 Children Act 1989) can be made that authorises a child assessment including a psychiatric assessment. There are additional powers available to the courts that include the making of an interim care order and care order. Harm includes impairment of health, which includes mental health (s.31 (9) Children Act 1989). This is important as the community care legislation in general does not apply to children or only applies in a qualified way.

It is important to realise that although considerable attention goes to the relatively small number of children who are at risk of being or who have actually been seriously abused, a much greater number of children have their development seriously challenged by adverse events, most of which are outside of their control or influence. These need to be considered by social workers and others. The speed of the changes is fast and the extent of the impact probably little appreciated by those who are not directly involved. Fortunately the relevant website permits close and detailed scrutiny and some free downloads of key documents is permitted.

One of the changes will be how services are organised and key to these is the establishment in most areas of Children's Trusts that will take the lead role in the coordination of local health, social care and education services as well as other agencies that may be working with children. This raises all sorts of issues about governance and even in some areas issues about geographical boundaries.

Figure 8.2 shows the various components that are required to keep focused on the child and the high level of integration needed, which will mean many agencies will have to rethink how they can engage in collaborative processes. Among the children

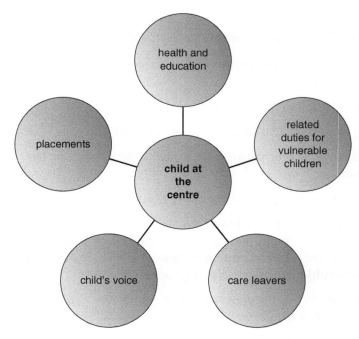

Figure 8.2   Keeping the child/young person at the centre

who have been identified as requiring a high degree of integrated services are those who have 'special circumstances', which includes children who are looked after; children of parents who experience mental health problems; and children who are exposed to domestic violence and family breakdown.

Although the government planned to remove the 'duty to cooperate' for schools and colleges this was retained and is still in place to give time for the reforms to embed. In October 2010 the heavily prescriptive statutory guidance on children's trusts were withdrawn and there was no longer a statutory requirement to produce a Children's and Young People's Plan but interestingly many still do.

One important initiative to safeguard children has been the **Common Assessment Framework** (CAF). This is a standardised approach to the assessment of a young person's needs and provides early indication of the requirement for services. This holistic assessment includes the role of parents, carers and the impact of external factors such as environment.

The CAF is a four-step process that assists practitioners to identify early on a young person's needs, assess those needs holistically, deliver coordinated services and review progress. It should be used when you are concerned about any aspect of how well a child or young person is progressing, or when a child or young person or parent/carer raises a concern, or when a child's or young person's needs are unclear, or broader than one individual service can satisfy.

The CAF process is voluntary so consent is needed and this means of course that some families will not want to engage with the process and that they can choose what information to share. The CAF is a request for services.

A **Team Around the Child** (TAC) is the team that has been established on a case-to-case basis to support the child, young person or family. The concept is that this team will enhance services by joined-up working, information sharing and early intervention. This can involve:

- a joined-up assessment, usually a Common Assessment Framework (CAF);
- a lead professional (LP) to coordinate the work;
- the child/young person and family at the centre of the process;
- a virtual or flexible multi-agency team that will change as needs change;
- coordination at the point of delivery;
- a TAC support plan to meet the needs of the child/young person;
- regular meetings to which the child/young person and families are invited to attend.

In some local areas the TAC is enlarged to become:

- a Team Around the Family (TAF) when dealing with families;
- a Team Around the School (TAS) where all the children with additional needs in a school are helped;
- a Team Around the House (TAH) when dealing with children in a home or facility.

This is delivered most effectively when one practitioner – a lead professional – takes a primary role to ensure frontline services are coordinated, coherent and achieving intended outcomes. Lead professionals are drawn from a range of professionals, not just social workers, and the process relies on the strength of relationship that this professional has established with the family, child or young person. This approach contrasts markedly when a child or young person may be assessed as requiring care and protection when they then become subject to child protection plans and only a qualified registered social worker can be the lead professional.

Information sharing is a key aspect of the above and raises some important issues for you to consider such as confidentiality and in general this should be dealt with on a case-to-case basis. It is important to remember there can be significant consequences to not sharing information as there can be to sharing information. You must use your professional judgement to decide whether to share or not, and what information is appropriate to share. Fortunately there is a helpful pocket guide to use and this can be accessed at the website **www.gov.uk**. (**https://media.education.gov.uk/assets/files/pdf/w/working%20together.pdf**)

(extract from **www.education.gov.uk/childrenandyoungpeople/strategy/integrated working/a0068944/team-around-the-child-tac**)

So far we have examined Inquiries to learn about when things go wrong and how the government is making a huge investment that should promote children and young people's life chances.

Does the separation of parents adversely affect the mental health of their children?

It is estimated that at least one in three children will experience parental separation before they reach the age of 16. Should this trend continue this would need to be looked on as the norm for families and we need to recognise that children need to learn coping skills that will better equip them to cope with these transitions. The research commissioned by JRF shows that no matter how well handled these separations might be they are difficult for children and young people to cope with. Although most will experience this as a period of unhappiness and distress that they work through, there are others who will struggle to cope with the effects that this has had on their lives. A small minority will experience mental health problems and some will need specialist help. In *Foundations* (2004) *Together and Apart* the JRF research shows among other highlights that the following are relevant:

- the quality of the parental relationship is important for the child's successful adjustment to post-separation circumstances;
- the older the child the more difficult it is to adjust to being in a stepfamily;
- extended families can play an important supportive role at the time of separation;
- at the time of separation the child's interests can be overlooked as a consequence of the preoccupation of the parental need;
- different children want different services, some like these to be at school and others want services that are outside of school.

However, children whose parents separate can benefit from the separation if it is handled well and it is much healthier to grow up in a reconstituted family that is at peace with each other than to remain in a family whose parents are continually at war with each other.

Problems that occur in the first few years

The risk of depression in mothers after childbirth (postpartum period) is greater than at any other time, with at least one woman in ten having a depressive episode within 12 months and the risk is greatest in the first three months after childbirth (Spender et al., 2001). Depression among adults has been covered in earlier chapters and we need to consider the impact on the child where the mother is distracted from the usual childrearing to deal with her own problems.

The cause of depression in mothers most likely has a biological component to it as does having a history of mental disorder, but once again social factors such as isolation, unemployment, lack of a confiding relationship, lack of supporting social networks are all factors that are likely to increase the risk of depression occurring. Childbirth is a major life event, mostly full of joy but also an event that requires a considerable change in lifestyle of the parent(s).

The impact on a mother and partner, if there is one, can be considerable and signs that would usually be picked up as possible indicators of depression can often be dismissed as simply the impact of a new baby. Depression needs to be distinguished from the onset of 'baby blues', which is very common and usually occurs in the first ten days but then goes, and depression, the onset of which is much later. There are numerous scales, such as the Edinburgh Postnatal Screening Depression Scale, that can be used to assess for depression. Health visitors and general practitioners should always be alert to this possibility, not least of which is being aware of the risk to the child in this situation.

RESEARCH EXAMPLE

In a programme developed with the Sainsbury Centre for Mental Health in Edinburgh, Staffordshire and Lewisham health visitors were trained to use a post-natal questionnaire and problem-solving skills. The impact of this training was evaluated using random control trials and the results suggest that the intervention was at least as effective as the use of anti-depressant medication.

(Sure Start, 2004)

Children's centres

Although Children's Centres have a wide remit including children's development, supporting parents especially in 'deprived communities', these centres also support children's health including mental health. Children's centres play a crucial role in early intervention and are intended to be the first port of call for families and carers who need help in order to tackle issues early and helping to prevent costly problems from emerging later on. Local authorities continue to have duties under the Childcare Act 2006 to consult before opening, closing or significantly changing children's centres, and to secure sufficient provision to meet local need so far as is reasonably practicable. Education and social services for children and young people are the responsibility of upper tier councils only (also known as county, metropolitan boroughs/cities, London boroughs and unitary authorities).

There are more than 3,600 children's centres in England although government financial cuts may bring about a reduction in provision under the objective of better targeting. They bring all the different support agencies together to offer a range of services, all in one place. There should be a children's centre in every community and centres in the most 'deprived' areas must provide a wider range of services including full day-care provision for children (minimum 10 hours a day). Centres serve around 800 children under five and the 'reach area' is intended to be within pram-pushing distance.

Children's centres in this way offer access to services that the target group generally does not use. This should help to address health inequalities especially with access to general practitioners, nurses and staff from specialist services such as community mental health and child and adolescent mental health services (CAMHS). Some centres have CAMHS workers seconded to them often on a part-time basis. What the centres try to achieve is improve mental health among children and their carers in a proactive rather than a reactive way.

Problems that occur in school age children

There are numerous behavioural problems that might beset some school age children. One of the difficult tasks is being able to differentiate between what in the present day is considered to be unruly or unusual behaviour and when that becomes a source of genuine concern as an indication of mental disorder. Not least of these is the somewhat controversial presence of attention deficit hyperactive disorder covered in Chapter 5.

Children whose parents have mental disorders

The effect on children who have at least one parent with a mental disorder is worthy of consideration. If we go back to the importance of stress as an intervening variable it is possible to realise the impact that mental disorder of a parent can have on the child caught in this situation. A study of 100 reviews of child deaths where abuse and neglect were factors showed that parental mental disorder was present in one-third of these cases (*Red Manual Code of Practice*, 2004).

Research carried out in the Netherlands examined the available literature and gathered together a panel of mental health practitioners all of whom had direct practice experience of working with children and their families (Rikken, 1995). They sought to identify what needed to be present to promote positive mental health. Out of this research came a number of findings including:

- the seriousness and chronicity of the parent's disorder was a significant factor;
- the quality of the relationship between the parent with mental disorder and the remaining parent was significant;
- the age and resilience of the child was an important variable; and
- the nature and extent of the social network to support the family.

The intervention in the Dutch project centred on work with the child and the 'healthy' parent, work to educate the family about the nature of the disorder and the development of social support networks. This is supported by other research showing that community-orientated and proactive initiatives are delivering measurable improvements in parenting skills (Lloyd, 1999; Walker, 2003).

Chapter 2 pulled together various factors that put people at risk of developing mental disorder. The impact on the children whose parents have mental disorder was described as being: problems at school, isolation and lack of specific information about their parent's mental disorder and prognosis. The outcome for children whose parent has a mental disorder will vary according to the severity of some of the variables mentioned earlier and will also depend upon the resilience and coping abilities of the child. However if a child grows up in a household where one of their parents has a chronic mental disorder they are at a greater risk of developing mental health problems than if their parent did not have a mental disorder.

This is considered to be so important that YoungMinds have suggested to the government that whenever an adult is diagnosed as experiencing a mental disorder, the law should require that the psychiatrist determines if that adult has parental responsibility for a child and if so that the psychiatrist has a duty to inform social services. This would allow extra support to be given to the family and child to mitigate against some of the negative factors surrounding their parent's mental disorder.

Of course there are other factors that can seriously disturb child development, such as having carers who abuse drugs, something that is becoming more and more common.

CASE EXAMPLE

Just as this manuscript was nearing completion in December 2013 a news story emerged worthy I think of inclusion in this chapter. This concerned Ms Alessandra Pachieri who is an Italian mother who gave birth by a caesarean section. She previously had two children who were born by C-section and whom are cared for by her family. That in itself is hardly unusual but Alessandra suffered from bipolar disorder and often had 'psychotic episodes'

(Continued)

(Continued)

and 'delusional beliefs'. This was the case when she had travelled to England in June 2012, to attend a training course at Stanstead airport and experienced a 'panic attack' that eventually resulted in her being compulsory admitted to a psychiatric hospital under the provisions of the Mental Health Act.

Ten weeks later in late August 2012 the NHS Trust caring for her took the unusual step of applying to the Court of Protection for a ruling to deliver her baby by a caesarean section against her will because the obstetricians treating her thought that allowing the mother a natural childbirth was to put both the mother and child in danger. The judge, Mr Justice Mostyn, at the Court of Protection ruled that at the time of the hearing that as she was one day from her due date and in his view she lacked capacity to make this decision, that the caesarean section would go ahead. The concern was that she would suffer a rupture to her womb.

At the same time Essex County Council began care proceedings which led to Alessandra's baby girl being eventually placed for adoption. This was reviewed in February 2013 by Britain's most senior judge, the president of the Family Division, Sir James Munby who ruled that the adoption could go ahead.

I am able to write about this as a High Court Judge refused a request from Essex County Council for a blanket ban on anything that could identify her. This in itself is unusual as the hearings in the Court of Protection are usually held in private to protect people who are judged not to have mental capacity and who are facing life or death decisions.

The released transcript of the Court of Protection judgement reveals 'that is, her mental health best interests', that the child be born alive and healthy and that result should be, if possible achieved, and such risks attendant should be avoided. 'I think, looked at her point of view, there is also a significant mental health advantage in her unborn child not being exposed to risk during his or her birth.' In those circumstances it seemed – 'and I very much hope restraint will not be necessary' – that the procedure that was proposed was 'manifestly in her best interests'. (5 December 2013 **www.localgovernmentlawyer.co.uk**/)

This has created a storm in both the UK and Italian national media, with claims that this was threatening to develop into an international row. Legally the adoption is safe but this may be one case where political imperatives results in the case being reconsidered. With 'freedom of movement' across the EU this opens up the prospect of further instances like this occurring between jurisdictions and may call for EU law to be enacted.

You are in the fortunate position of being able to see how this turned out.

Small child but big worries

New developments in child mental health indicate that depression and anxiety can be present in very young children. The rationale for this lies in the concept that we all carry with us a genetic predisposition to psychological problems. This is in itself is not so contentious but the idea that this can be triggered as early as the first year of life certainly is; although we have recognised that babies, infants and toddlers differ from one another in behaviour the idea that this can extend to mental health is new.

A non-profit child advocacy group in the USA by the name of 'ZerotoThree' estimates that up to 10% of very young children have some kind of 'clinical condition' and makes the point that this may set up concerns about mental health and disorder for later life. One of the difficulties that we have of course is that babies cannot talk or at least, even as they develop, have the vocabulary that allows for the expression of issues of anxiety and depression. However we can infer from the ways that babies play that they are happy or distressed and similarly we can look at the way in which carers and babies interact. We do know that the first three years in particular of development are crucial to establish the sort of person that we will develop into and the type of relationships that we will develop. For further information about this work consult Zerotothree's website **www.zerotothree. org/about-us/zero-to-thees-fact-sheet.html**

Safeguarding children in whom illness is fabricated or induced

A Department of Health Guidance document for Children's Safeguarding Boards recognised that children may be at risk as a result of their carer attempting to have them diagnosed with some form of illness. Here we see played out a familiar tension referred to by the earlier information from the Lords Hansard about how to protect children from real but rare events, while not wrongly accusing carers of deliberate attempts to harm the children in their care.

There are four main ways that the carer may fabricate or induce illness in a child. These include:

- signs and symptoms;

- falsification of medical records;

- falsification of bodily fluids and/or letters or records; and

- induction of illness by different means.

(adapted from DoH, 2001)

It is important to realise that while as a social worker you should be aware of this phenomenon and alert when vulnerable people are at risk, the diagnosis of this disorder needs to be left with specialists who are experienced and have training in this type of diagnosis.

Understanding children

Sally Gorin at the NSPCC has carried out a literature review that draws together evidence about how children have experienced living with domestic violence, parental substance abuse and parental ill health, both physical and mental. This can make some children very vulnerable and in need of support. The themes that emerged included:

- children are much more aware of their parent's problems than the parents imagined which in turn can lead to high levels of concern about their parent's safety;

- children tend to use informal support and talk to either parents, siblings or friends;

- when they did go to professionals they were not always satisfied with their contact and felt that they were not listened to, whereas what they wanted was someone to listen to them and in whom they could place their trust;

- age-appropriate information was needed to help children to understand what is going on in their family.

(Adapted from Gorin in *Findings*, 2004, JRF)

The following gives a good picture of what the experience must be like and how children feel.

> *Sadness and isolation that children may experience can be perpetuated by the stigma and secrecy that surrounds domestic violence, parental substance misuse and ill health. Some children report feeling depressed, having problems making or maintaining friends, having a disrupted education or experiencing bullying.*

(*Findings*, May 2004, p.2)

Not all children suffer long-term effects and they are often very resilient and bounce back from these adverse conditions.

Assessment of risk and resilience

It is commonly thought that when children are exposed to adverse and stressful situations their mental health will suffer. This is in spite of evidence that suggests that there is not a causal relationship. Clearly in a relatively small number of instances children are at immediate risk of serious harm and the numerous Inquiries where this was overlooked make sobering reading. However, it is also the case that many, many more children experience turmoil and adversity in their lives and not only survive it but actually do well. Is it possible that in concentrating upon the individual risk, for all the right reasons, we might overlook the positive effect that social factors might make to help the individuals cope with adversity? Have we got the balance right between protecting children from risk and promoting in them the ability to bounce back when they experience difficulties? Certain key factors crop up time and time again when we look at how some people experience distress and cope. These are described by the term resilience.

Resilience has a near-universal meaning to it and is best summed up as:

> *Resilient children are better equipped to resist stress and adversity, cope with change and uncertainty, and to recover faster and more completely from traumatic events or episodes.*

(Newman and Blackburn, 2001, p.1)

There is extensive documentation of both risk and resilience in the social science and social work literature (Rutter, 1999; Walker, 2003; 2011) and the common factors that can be deduced fit well into the schematic chart that was presented in Chapter 2. If we take the main headings used in the chart we can list the following factors:

Social causation factors
- having a strong extended family;
- successful schooling;
- network of friends;
- having a role outside of the family – volunteering, sports, clubs;
- member of a religious community.

Psychological factors
- warm, supportive carers;
- good parent–child relationships;
- parental harmony;
- confiding relationship with at least one parent.

Personal
- age;
- higher IQ;
- social skills;
- humour;
- temperament.

(Adapted from Newman and Blackburn, 2002)

However, where the above are not present and replaced by low income/poverty, over-involved parents and social exclusion then the child's ability to bounce back from adverse and stressful events is much less likely to occur. Although as social workers we are often involved in short-term crisis resolution, the most damaging impact on child development is most likely to be where the situation is chronic and with little prospect of improvement.

A psycho-social educational approach with parents

ACTIVITY 8.2

What strategies could be adopted in order to help children to cope better and develop resilience? Write down what you think could be done and by whom. Spend a few minutes on this task.

(Continued)

(Continued)

COMMENT

It ought to help if you refer to Figure 2.1 that was used in Chapter 2. This will give you direct clues about where the need might be but this tool is better at analysis rather than strategy. What works for children coping with adverse situations is having the support of their extended family, neighbours or mentors and having close friends in whom to confide, rather than the specific activities of professionals (Newman and Blackburn, 2002). How different was this to your ideas? Should the social work task be one of mobilising community support, supporting, befriending and building up a database for service users to make contact with each other? Children need to have opportunities to learn coping skills in the face of difficult situations. They need to develop self-esteem and to feel valued if not at home then outside of the home. Social workers and others should always look to the strengths as well as the problems in each individual's situation.

Empowering intervention

The psycho-social model of intervention provides a conceptual tool for social workers to work with the diverse populations that make up the UK.

ACTIVITY 8.3

As a social worker working with Asian children you realise that they are trying to respond to their parents' cultural practices when at home and to the cultural norms of their white friends when at school. As they are getting older the tension between the two is becoming more apparent and their behaviour at school is becoming a problem. The teachers at the local school have asked you to give some advice to them. What would be your response?

COMMENT

Of course there is no easy answer. The use of the psycho-social model allows you to conceptualise some of the problems and to see them as potentially having an adverse impact on the children's development. You are trying to work anti-oppressively but just who is your client? What cultural norms would you respect?

Evidence-based practice

How do we know what works, why it works and with whom it works best? These questions should be at the heart of the reflective practitioner and throughout this book an attempt has been made to locate practice alongside evidence. If social work is to stand alongside other professions we must be able to support our claim with evidence that what we do actually works.

There are a number of information systems that provide up-to-date research reports about mental health and other work with service users. Facilities such as the Cochrane Library, The NHS Centre for Reviews and Dissemination and the Social Care Institute for Excellence (SCIE) provide academics, students and practitioners with electronic forms of data and research evaluations. An excellent text written by Martin Weber is *Evidence-based Policy and Practice in Mental Health Social Work* in this series. But this on its own is insufficient and social workers will need to enhance their own evaluative and research skills in order to make best practice common practice.

CHAPTER SUMMARY

This chapter has drawn together the idea of working together to provide the kind of effective mental health service that service users want and that will provide children with care and protection. Social workers can be involved as members of a team that responds to the needs of users including children. Children need to be more involved not just with their care and treatment but also should be consulted about service design and delivery. That they are not says more about our lack of imagination and faith than their abilities.

Child protection can never be far away from social work discourse and two Inquiries were considered to demonstrate what happens when things go wrong. Children also need to be recognised as potentially strong and resilient and the social work role might well be to enhance these strengths rather than concentrate on weaknesses. It is a reality that many children experience trauma and loss and work through this transition and emerge relatively unscathed.

Using the psycho-social model of intervention, various ways of working with parents were addressed and the advantage of this to social workers is that it allows us to make full use of a holistic view of mental disorder.

FURTHER READING

Clothier, C. (1994) *The Allitt Inquiry* considered the Beverly Allitt case, answering such questions as how she was allowed to qualify as a nurse, why her crimes were not detected sooner and what can be done to prevent another similar tragedy occurring in the future? The Inquiry also makes recommendations for changes in procedures.

Newman, T. and Blackburn, S. (2002) of Barnardo's Policy, Research and influencing Unit have produced a must-read paper that provides an in-depth examination of many of the issues raised in this chapter. It is called *Transitions in the Lives of Children and Young People: Resilience factors*, published by the Scottish Executive Education Department and available electronically. **www.scotland.gov.uk/ publications**

Spender, Q., Salt, N., Dawkins, J., Kendrick, T. and Hill, P. (2001) *Child Mental Health in Primary Care*. Abingdon: Radcliffe Medical Press is an excellent text that covers numerous child mental health problems and more. Includes check-lists and assessment questionnaires.

The booklet Principles for Practice (contains the Circle of involvement)ideas and more can be obtained from the Trent Multi Professional Deanery by emailing Rachel.Hawley@tsha.nhs.uk

Webber, M. (2011) *Evidence-based Policy and Practice in Mental Health Social Work (Second edition).* Exeter: Learning Matters.

WEBSITES

www.nhsdirect.nhs.uk

www.mind.org.uk www.sane.org.uk

www.nsf.org.uk www.doh.gov.uk/mentalhealth

www.bbc.co.uk/health/mental/

MACA (Mental Aftercare Association) maca.bs@maca.org.uk **www.maca.org.uk**

Parenting Plus **www.parentlineplus.org.uk**

Winston's Wish info@winstonswish.org.uk **www.winstonswish.org.uk**

Social Care institute for Excellence **www.scie.org.uk**

Young Minds enquiries@youngminds.org.uk **www.youngminds.org.uk**

Lords Hansard **www.publication.parliament.uk**

All JRF Findings are published on their website: **www.jrf.org.uk**

Glossary

Approved Clinician (AC) This is an important new role that is not restricted to doctors and could include social workers. ACs have some of the powers that previously were reserved for doctors; this includes holding an inpatient for up to 72 hours in hospital to allow an application for assessment to be made.

Approved Doctor under s.12 of the 1983 Mental Health Act A s.12 doctor is approved by the Secretary of State as 'having special experience in the diagnosis and treatment of mental disorder'. Each region has its own selection panel, which sets standards for doctors who seek approval in their area.

Approved Mental Health Professional (AMHP) Section 118 of the MHA 2007 sees the role of the ASW replaced with the new role of AMHP. Only the AMHP or the nearest relative can make an application for compulsory admission. Unlike the ASW role, the AMHP may be drawn from a range of professionals, not doctors, but includes registered social workers, first-level nurses, occupational therapists or chartered psychologists.

Approved Social Worker (ASW) A qualified social worker who has undergone a 12-week additional training course. In order to comply with the 1983 Mental Health Act and ensure their independence, the ASW must be appointed and employed by the Local Social Services Department. Most ASWs transferred to the new role of Approved Mental Health Professional in October 2008. After this point the role of ASW will be of historical note only.

Behaviour modification Based on the idea of learning theory and conditioning. Intervention focuses on the relearning of behaviour.

Best Interest Assessors (BIA) This is a new role that provides an assessment to ensure that any act or decision made for or on behalf of a person who lacks capacity is made in his/her best interests.

BNF Stands for the **British National Formulary** reference text, which is published twice a year and contains up-to-date information about the maximum dosage of medication for patients. Hospital wards should always have the latest copy available.

Bolam test Where a healthcare professional is not considered to be negligent if s/he adopts the practice which a responsible body of professionals (e.g. psychiatrists, nurses or social workers) accept as appropriate.

CAMHS Child and Adolescent Mental Health Services.

Care Quality Commission (CQC) The independent regulator of health care and adult social care services in England. They also protect the interests of patients whose rights have been restricted under the Mental Health Act.

CMHT Community Mental Health Team.

Cognitive therapy A treatment intervention, available on the NHS, that focuses on maladaptive patterns of thinking that affect the person's behaviour.

Court of Protection Part VII of the 1983 Mental Health Act aims to protect the property and financial affairs of an individual who is incapable of acting because of a mental disorder. The MHA also provides safeguards for anyone authorised by the Court of Protection to manage the patient's finances.

CPN Community psychiatric nurses are qualified and experienced psychiatric nurses who play a major role in the supervision and treatment of patients in the community. Along with ASWs, psychiatrists and others, they have a pivotal role in community mental health and outreach teams.

CSIP NIMHE (National Institute of Mental Health for England) has now been absorbed into a successor body Care Services Improvement Partnership (CSIP). CSIP embraces eight programmes. They are the National Child and Adolescent Mental Health Services (CAMHS) Support Service; Health in Criminal Justice; the Integrated Care Network; Integrating Community Equipment and Support; the National Institute for Mental Health in England; the Health and Social Care Change Agent Team; the Valuing People Support Team; and Children for Change. It has an annual budget of more than £30 million. Chief executive: Richard Humphries. Website: **www.csip.org.uk**

Deprivation of liberty safeguards (DoLS) Section 50 of the MHA has amended the MCA 2005 to provide safeguards for those incapable people over 18 years of age that are deprived of liberty.

Diagnosis Forms part of the assessment process and the identification of specific mental disorder in which reference is made to either the **DSM IV** or to the **ICD–10** reference texts, both of which classify mental disorder.

Expressed emotion This term is used usually in the sense that the family may have 'high expressed emotion' that is having an adverse effect on the service user. This includes over-involved parents and a highly critical atmosphere.

Family therapy The focus is on working with the family to restore the family system to a more functioning unit.

Health Care Professions Council (HCPC) formerly the Health Professions Council is a statutory regulator of social work, nursing and other professions. Qualified social workers are able to apply to go onto the register and thus be able to call themselves by the legal title of social worker.

Home Office Mental Health Unit The Mental Health Unit was formerly known as C3 Division and it exercises the Home Secretary's powers in respect of restricted patients under the 1983 MHA.

HSC Health service circular.

HSG Health service guidance.

Independent Mental Capacity Advocates (IMCAs) provide a specialist advocacy service for people who lack capacity and who have no one, other than paid staff, to support them.

LA Local authority.

LAC Local Authority Circular.

LSSA Local Social Services Authority in England.

Mental Health Act (MHA) 1983 Although this legislation is over 20 years old it is still the primary legislation in this area. It is primarily about the compulsory admission, treatment and discharge of people who are diagnosed as having a mental disorder.

Mental Health Act (MHA) 2007 The main purpose of the 2007 Act is to amend the 1983 Act. It also introduces 'deprivation of liberty safeguards' through amending the Mental Capacity Act 2005 (MCA); supervised community treatment orders and extends the rights of victims by amending the Domestic Violence, Crime and Victims Act 2004. The main purpose of the legislation has been redefined to ensure that people with serious mental disorders and which threaten **either** their health or safety **or** the safety of the public can be treated even if they object if it is considered necessary to prevent them from harming themselves or others.

Mental Health Act Commission (MHAC) was effectively transferred to the Care Quality Commission which will provide an integrated approach to regulation of the sector.

Mental Health Act (MHA) hospital managers For the purposes of the 1983 Mental Health Act (MHA) it is important to differentiate between 'MHA managers' and any other hospital staff who may also be referred to as 'managers' in terms of a general management structure, e.g. a directorate manager or CMHT manager is not the 'MHA manager' in respect of the MHA. It is the 'MHA managers' who are the formal detaining authority under the Act, not the registered medical practitioner/responsible medical officer (RMO). At common law, 'the managers/NHS Trust' … are legally liable for any deprivation of liberty which is not justified by the Act.

Mental Health Act (MHA) Hospital Managers' Review Patients who are detained in hospital may request that the reasons for their continued detention in hospital are reviewed by the MHA hospital managers. The MHA hospital managers (s.23) can order the discharge of an unrestricted detained patient.

Mental Health Review Tribunal has now been superseded by a **First-tier Tribunal**.

Mental Health Tribunal/First-tier Tribunal The First-tier Tribunal (Mental Health) often called the **Mental Health Tribunal** hears applications from people detained under the Mental Health Act 1983 (as amended by the Mental Health Act 2007) and replaces the Mental Health Review Tribunal. This is the 'court' which convenes at the hospital at which the patient is detained and which determines whether the grounds for detention under the Act continue to exist. The panel consists of three members: the medical member, usually a consultant psychiatrist, a legal member (a lawyer, often a judge in restricted cases), and a lay member.

The jurisdiction covers the whole of England. Wales has a separate provision. The Tribunal sits within the Health, Education and Social Care Chamber of the First-tier Tribunal.

National Institute for Clinical Excellence (NICE) Conducts research and evaluations of various treatments and publishes guidance and advice.

Nearest relative (NR) Clearly defined under s.26 of the MHA 1983.The nearest relative (NR) is usually, but not always, the patient's next-of-kin. Section 26 explains how to identify the NR. A common mnemonic is '**How Should Folk be Graded, Give Us NewS**'. That is, **h**usband/wife; **s**on/daughter; **f**ather/mother; **b**rother/sister; **g**randparents; **g**randchild; **u**ncle/aunt; **n**ephew/niece; **s**ame sex partner. If the relatives are of equal standing, the eldest is preferred. In-laws are usually excluded. The patient cannot choose who the NR should be. It is now the case that in the case of civil partners, one will be the nearest relative of the other regardless of the time they have lived together.

National Institute of Mental Health England (NIMHE) See Care Services Improvement Partnership (CSIP).

NHS National Health Service.

Patient The term used throughout the MHA as is the male pronoun. Social workers use the term service user, implying more of a partnership exists between themselves and the 'user' of the service but patient is still used in the hospital setting.

The Mental Health Act 1983 provides that, unless otherwise stated and except in relation to the Court of Protection, the word *patient* means 'a person suffering or appearing to suffer from a mental disorder' (s.145(1)). In the context of tribunal proceedings, the patient is simply the person whose case is under review. There are a number of different types of patients, e.g. informal patients, voluntary patients and restricted patients.

PCT Primary Care Trust.

PGO The Public Guardianship Office which is the executive agency based in the Lord Chancellor's office and which carries out the work of the Court of Protection.

PHCT Primary health care team.

Prognosis The medical assessment of the future course of events and probable outcome of the patient's mental disorder.

Psychoanalysis Based on Freud, the aim is through the client/therapist relationship to resolve conflicted states of mind. Not available on the NHS.

Responsible Clinician (RC) This new role replaces the responsible medical officer (RMO) who until the Mental Health Act 2007 was the doctor who had full legal and clinical responsibility for a detained patient. Providing that the RC has already undertaken training as an AC, he/she need not be a doctor.

Responsible Medical Officer (RMO) The psychiatrist who has full clinical and legal responsibility for a patient detained under the 1983 Mental Health Act. Described within the 1983 MHA as the doctor who is in charge of the treatment of the patient.

They will usually be a consultant psychiatrist and approved under s.12 of the MHA as having a special experience in the diagnosis and treatment of mental disorder. Due to be replaced by the RC.

Second Opinion Appointed Doctor (SOAD) A registered medical practitioner (experienced psychiatrist) appointed by the MHAC to provide an independent opinion in respect of Consent to Treatment under Part IV of the 1983 Mental Health Act.

Section 12 Approved Doctor Approved by the Secretary of State as '... *having special experience in the diagnosis and treatment of mental disorder*'. Each strategic health authority/region has its own selection panel which sets standards for doctors who seek approval in their area, receives and scrutinises applications and grants approval under the 1983 MHA where appropriate.

SHA Special Health Authority.

SSD Social Services Department.

Statutory A requirement dictated by Act of Parliament, e.g. the 1983 Mental Health Act.

Statutory duty A duty that must be complied with if contained within an Act of Parliament.

Statutory instrument Relates to delegated legislation drafted by the relevant department under powers attributed by an Act of Parliament. Statutory regulations are most commonly drafted as Statutory instruments and laid before Parliament, e.g. The Mental Health (Hospital, Guardianship and Consent to Treatment) Regulations 1983.

Appendix 1

Professional capabilities framework

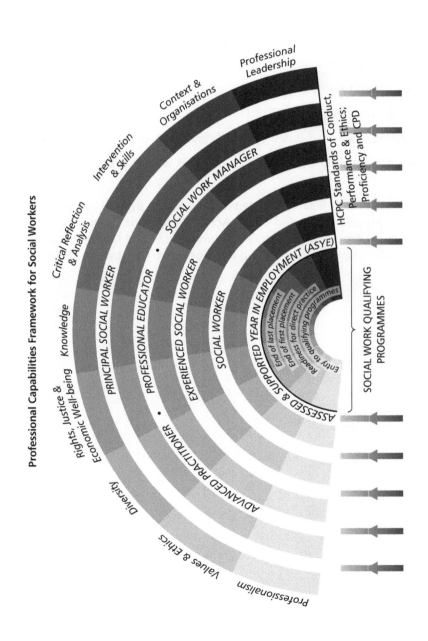

Professional Capabilities Framework for Social Workers

Professional Leadership

Context & Organisations

Intervention & Skills

Critical Reflection & Analysis

Knowledge

Rights, Justice & Economic Well-being

Diversity

Values & Ethics

Professionalism

PRINCIPAL SOCIAL WORKER

PROFESSIONAL EDUCATOR

EXPERIENCED SOCIAL WORKER

SOCIAL WORKER

SOCIAL WORK MANAGER

ADVANCED PRACTITIONER

ASSESSED & SUPPORTED YEAR IN EMPLOYMENT (ASYE)

End of last placement

End of first placement

Readiness for direct practice

Entry to qualifying programmes

HCPC Standards of Conduct, Performance & Ethics; Proficiency and CPD

SOCIAL WORK QUALIFYING PROGRAMMES

Appendix 2
Subject benchmark for social work

Defining principles

4.1 As an applied academic subject, social work is characterised by a distinctive focus on practice in complex social situations to promote and protect individual and collective well-being. This underscores the importance of partnerships between HEIs and service providers to ensure the full involvement of practitioners, managers, tutors, service users and carers with students in both academic and practice learning and assessment.

4.2 At honours level, the study of social work involves the integrated study of subject-specific knowledge, skills and values and the critical application of research knowledge from the social and human sciences, and from social work (and closely related domains) to inform understanding and to underpin action, reflection and evaluation. Honours degree programmes should be designed to help foster this integration of contextual, analytic, critical, explanatory and practical understanding.

4.3 Contemporary definitions of social work as a degree subject reflect its origins in a range of different academic and practice traditions. The precise nature and scope of the subject is itself a matter for legitimate study and critical debate. Three main issues are relevant to this.

- Social work is located within different social welfare contexts. Within the UK there are different traditions of social welfare (influenced by legislation, historical development and social attitudes) and these have shaped both social work education and practice in community-based settings including residential, day care and substitute care. In an international context, distinctive national approaches to social welfare policy, provision and practice have greatly influenced the focus and content of social work degree programmes.

- There are competing views in society at large on the nature of social work and on its place and purpose. Social work practice and education inevitably reflect these differing perspectives on the role of social work in relation to social justice, social care and social order.

- Social work, both as occupational practice and as an academic subject, evolves, adapts and changes in response to the social, political and economic challenges and demands of contemporary social welfare policy, practice and legislation.

4.6 Social work is a moral activity that requires practitioners to recognise the dignity of the individual, but also to make and implement difficult decisions (including restriction of liberty) in human situations that involve the potential for benefit or harm.

Honours degree programmes in social work therefore involve the study, application of, and critical reflection upon, ethical principles and dilemmas. As reflected by the four care councils' codes of practice, this involves showing respect for persons, honouring the diverse and distinctive organisations and communities that make up contemporary society, promoting social justice and combating processes that lead to discrimination, marginalisation and social exclusion. This means that honours undergraduates must learn to:

- recognise and work with the powerful links between intrapersonal and interpersonal factors and the wider social, legal, economic, political and cultural context of people's lives;
- understand the impact of injustice, social inequalities and oppressive social relations;
- challenge constructively individual, institutional and structural discrimination;
- practise in ways that maximise safety and effectiveness in situations of uncertainty and incomplete information;
- help people to gain, regain or maintain control of their own affairs, insofar as this is compatible with their own or others' safety, well-being and rights;
- work in partnership with service users and carers and other professionals to foster dignity, choice and independence, and effect change.

4.7 The expectation that social workers will be able to act effectively in such complex circumstances requires that honours degree programmes in social work should be designed to help students learn to become accountable, reflective, critical and evaluative. This involves learning to:

- think critically about the complex social, legal, economic, political and cultural contexts in which social work practice is located;
- work in a transparent and responsible way, balancing autonomy with complex, multiple and sometimes contradictory accountabilities (for example, to different service users, employing agencies, professional bodies and the wider society);
- exercise authority within complex frameworks of accountability and ethical and legal boundaries;
- acquire and apply the habits of critical reflection, self-evaluation and consultation, and make appropriate use of research in decision-making about practice and in the evaluation of outcomes.

Subject knowledge, understanding and skills
Subject knowledge and understanding

5.1 During their degree studies in social work, honours graduates should acquire, critically evaluate, apply and integrate knowledge and understanding in the following five core areas of study.

5.1.1 Social work services, service users and carers, which include:
- the social processes (associated with, for example, poverty, migration, unemployment, poor health, disablement, lack of education and other sources of disadvantage) that

lead to marginalisation, isolation and exclusion, and their impact on the demand for social work services;

- explanations of the links between definitional processes contributing to social differences (for example, social class, gender, ethnic differences, age, sexuality and religious belief) to the problems of inequality and differential need faced by service users;

- the nature of social work services in a diverse society (with particular reference to concepts such as prejudice, interpersonal, institutional and structural discrimination, empowerment and anti-discriminatory practices);

- the nature and validity of different definitions of, and explanations for, the characteristics and circumstances of service users and the services required by them, drawing on knowledge from research, practice experience, and from service users and carers;

- the focus on outcomes, such as promoting the well-being of young people and their families, and promoting dignity, choice and independence for adults receiving services;

- the relationship between agency policies, legal requirements and professional boundaries in shaping the nature of services provided in interdisciplinary contexts and the issues associated with working across professional boundaries and within different disciplinary groups.

5.1.2 *The service delivery context, which includes:*
- the location of contemporary social work within historical, comparative and global perspectives, including European and international contexts;

- the changing demography and cultures of communities in which social workers will be practising;

- the complex relationships between public, social and political philosophies, policies and priorities and the organisation and practice of social work, including the contested nature of these;

- the issues and trends in modern public and social policy and their relationship to contemporary practice and service delivery in social work;

- the significance of legislative and legal frameworks and service delivery standards (including the nature of legal authority, the application of legislation in practice, statutory accountability and tensions between statute, policy and practice);

- the current range and appropriateness of statutory, voluntary and private agencies providing community-based, day-care, residential and other services and the organisational systems inherent within these;

- the significance of interrelationships with other related services, including housing, health, income maintenance and criminal justice (where not an integral social service).

5.1.3 *Values and ethics, which include:*
- the nature, historical evolution and application of social work values;

- the moral concepts of rights, responsibility, freedom, authority and power inherent in the practice of social workers as moral and statutory agents;

- the complex relationships between justice, care and control in social welfare and the practical and ethical implications of these, including roles as statutory agents and in upholding the law in respect of discrimination;

- aspects of philosophical ethics relevant to the understanding and resolution of value dilemmas and conflicts in both interpersonal and professional contexts;

- the conceptual links between codes defining ethical practice, the regulation of professional conduct and the management of potential conflicts generated by the codes held by different professional groups.

5.1.4 Social work theory, which includes:
- research-based concepts and critical explanations from social work theory and other disciplines that contribute to the knowledge base of social work, including their distinctive epistemological status and application to practice;

- the relevance of sociological perspectives to understanding societal and structural influences on human behaviour at individual, group and community levels;

- the relevance of psychological, physical and physiological perspectives to understanding personal and social development and functioning.

5.1.5 The nature of social work practice, which includes:
- the characteristics of practice in a range of community-based and organisational settings within statutory, voluntary and private sectors, and the factors influencing changes and developments in practice within these contexts.

References

Ahmed, B. (1991) *Interpreters in Public Services* (eds Baker, P, Hussain, Z and Saunders, J). Birmingham: Venture Press.

Alcock, J. (2003) *Mental Health Services – Workforce design and development – best practice guidance.* London: DoH.

American Psychiatric Association (1994) *Diagnostic and Statistical Manual of Mental Disorders (DSM–IV).* Washington DC: American Psychiatric Association.

Archanbeault, J. (2009) *Reflective Reader: Social Work and Mental Health.* Learning Matters: Exeter.

Arnstein, S. (1969) A ladder of citizen participation in the USA. *Journal of the American Institute of Planners,* Vol 35, no 4.

Banks, S. (2002) *Ethics and Values in Social Work.* Basingstoke: Macmillan.

Bartlett, P. and Sandland, R. (2003) *Mental Health Law, Policy and Practice.* Oxford: Oxford University Press.

Bean, P. (1986) *Mental Disorder and Legal Control.* Cambridge: Cambridge University Press.

Bhopal, R. Spectre of racism in health and health care: lessons from history and the United States. *British Medical Journal,* 27 June 1998; 316: 1970–1973.

Blackburn, D. and Golightley, M. (2004) European Sociological Conference paper. University of Lincoln.

Bland, R. (2009) *Social Work Practice in Mental Health: an introduction.* Australia: Allen and Unwin.

Bowers, L., Clark, N. and Callaghan, P. (2003) Multidisciplinary reflections on assessment for compulsory admission: the views of Approved Social Workers, general practitioners, ambulance crews, police, community psychiatric nurses and psychiatrists. *British Journal of Social Work,* Vol. 33, 961–8.

Brammer, A. (2003) *Social Work Law.* Harlow: Pearson Educational.

Braye, S. Preston-Shoot, M. et al. (2005) *Teaching, Learning and Assessment of Law in Social Work Education.* Bristol: SCIE. Bristol: Policy Press.

Brock, A. and Griffiths, C. (2003) *Trends in the Mortality of Young Adults Aged 15–44 in England and Wales 1961–2001.* Office of National Statistics: Health Statistics Quarterly. See also website: **www. statistics.gov.uk**

Brown, G.W. and Harris, T.O. (1978) *The Social Origins of Depression.* London: Tavistock.

Brown, R. and Barber, P. (2008) *The Social Worker's Guide to Mental Capacity Law.* Exeter: Learning Matters.

Butler, A. and Pritchard, C. (1983) *Social Work and Mental Illness.* Basingstoke: Macmillan.

Burns, T., Knapp, M., Catty, J., Healey, A., Henderson, J., Watt, H. et al. (2001) Home treatment for mental health problems: a systematic review. *Health Technology Assessment,* 5 (15).

Burns, T. (2013) Community treatment orders for patients with psychosis (OCTET): a randomised controlled trial. *The Lancet,* 381 (9878), 1627–633, 11 May 2013.

Campbell (1999) *Training for Mental Health 3: Exploring key areas.* Brighton: Pavilion Publishing.

Campbell, J. in K. O'Hagan (ed.) *Competence in Social Work Practice: A practical guide for professionals.* London: Routledge, Kegan Paul.

Care Services Improvement (2006) *Reviewing the Care Programme Approach 2006: A consultation document.* London: CSI.

Care Quality Commission (March 2011) *Patients experiences of the First-tier Tribunal (Mental Health) Report of a joint pilot project of the Administrative Justice & Tribunals Council and the Care Quality Commission* at **www.cqc.org.uk/sites/default/files/media/documents/pe_first_tier_tribunal_report. pdf**

Carpenter, J., Schneider, J., Brandon, T. and Wooff, D. (2003) Working in multidisciplinary mental health teams: the impact on social workers and health professionals of integrated mental health care. *British Journal of Social Work,* 33, 1081–103.

Clark, C. (2000) *Social Work Ethics.* Basingstoke: Macmillan.

Clothier, C. (1994) *Report of the Inquiry into Beverley Allit: The Allit Inquiry* (1991). London: HMSO.

Cochrane, R. (1983) *The Social Creation of Mental Illness.* London: Longman Applied Psychology.

Coid, J.W. (1996) Dangerous patients with mental illness; increased risks warrant new policies, adequate resources, and appropriate legislation. *British Medical Journal,* 312, 965–6.

Community Care (2012) *Where social workers are going wrong on the Mental Capacity Act* at **www. communitycare.co.uk/2012/10/30/where-social-workers-are-going-wrong-on-the-mental-capacity-act**

Community Care (2013) *Practice Standards for BIA* accessed 21/10/2013 at **www.communitycare. co.uk/practice-standards-for -best-interests-assessors-launched**

Coulshed, V. (1991) *Social Work Practice: An Introduction.* Basingstoke: Macmillan.

Crawford, K. and Walker, J. (2003) *Social Work and Human Development.* Exeter: Learning Matters.

Cree, V. (2002) The changing nature of social work in R. Adams et al. (eds) *Social Work: Themes, issues and critical debates.* Basingstoke: Palgrave.

Curran, C. and Grimshaw, C. (2000) Consent to treatment for medication under the 1983 Mental Health Act. *Openmind,* March/April, No 102, 24–5.

Curran, C., Grimshaw, C. and Hewitt, D. (2001) The Human Rights Act and mental health law. *Openmind,* May June, No 109, 24–5.

Curran, C., Golightley, M. and Fennell, P. (2014) Social Circumstances Reports for Mental health tribunals, **Legal Action** Part 1 March 2014 Part 2tba.

Curran, C., Grimshaw, C. and Zigmond, A. (1997) The doctor's holding power under section 5(2) *Openmind,* No 83, 28.

Deegan, P. (1996) Coping with recovery as a journey of the heart. *Psychiatric Rehabilitation Journal,* Vol 19, no 3. Also at **http://shrp.rutgers.edu/dept/psyr/employment/documents/1996PatriciaDeegan Article.pdf**

Dein , S. (1997) Clinical review. ABC of mental health: mental health in a multiethnic society. *British Medical Journal.*

Department for Children, Schools and Families (DCSF)(2008) *Children's Plan Targeted Mental Health in Schools (TaMHS)* at **http://webarchive.nationalarchives.gov.uk/20130401151715/ www.education.gov.uk/publications/**

Department for Constitutional Affairs (2007) *Mental Capacity Act 2005 Code of Practice.* Issued by the Lord Chancellor on 23 April 2007 in accordance with sections 42 and 43 of the Act. London: TSO.

Department of Health (1990) *National Health Service and Community Care Act.* London: DoH.

Department of Health (1993) *The Health of the Nation: A strategy for health in England.* London: HMSO.

Department of Health (1995) *Building Bridges Report.* London: DoH.

Department of Health (1995) *A Handbook on Child and Adolescent Mental Health.* London: HMSO.

Department of Health (1998) *Modernising Mental Health Services: National Priorities Guidance 1999/00–2001/02* LAC(98)22.

Department of Health (1998) *Modernising Mental Health Services: Safe, sound and supportive.* London: DoH.

Department of Health (1998) *Partnerships in Action: New opportunities for joint working between health and social services: a discussion document.* London: DoH.

Department of Health (1999) *Code of Practice to the Mental Health Act 1983 (revised 1999).* Norwich: Stationery Office.

Department of Health (1999) *Effective Care Co-Ordination in Mental Health Services: Modernising the Care Programme Approach – a policy booklet.* London: DoH.

Department of Health (1999) *National Service Framework for Mental Health – Modern Standards and Service Models.* London: DoH.

Department of Health (1999) *Quality Protects Programme: Transforming children's services 2000–01* LAC (99) 33, London: HMSO.

Department of Health (1999) *The Mental Health Act 1983 Revised Code of Practice.* London: DoH.

Department of Health (1999) *Safer Services: National confidential inquiry into suicide and homicide by people with mental illness.* London: DoH.

Department of Health (2000) *The NHS Plan: a plan for investment: a plan for reform.* London: HMSO.

Department of Health (2001) *Safeguarding Children in Whom Illness is Induced or Fabricated by Carers with Parenting Responsibilities.* London: HMSO.

Department of Health (2001) *Treatment Choice in Psychological Therapies and Counselling: Evidence based clinical practice guidelines.* London: DoH.

Department of Health (2001) *The Mental Health Policy Implementation Guide.* London: DoH.

Department of Health (2001) *Valuing People: A new strategy for learning disability for the 21st century.* London: TSO.

Department of Health (2002) *A Sign of the Times: Modernising mental health services for people who are deaf.* London: DoH.

Department of Health (2002) *Dual Diagnosis Good Practice Guide.* London: TSO.

Department of Health (2002) *Mental Health Implementation Guide: Dual diagnosis good practice guide.* London: DoH.

Department of Health (2003) *Delivering Race Equality: A Framework for Action.* Consultation Document. London: DoH.

Department of Health (2003) *Skills for Health.* London: DoH.

Department of Health (2003) *Women's Mental Health: Into the mainstream: strategic development of mental health care for women.* London: DoH.

Department of Health (2004) *An Easy Guide to Direct Payments.* London: TSO.

Department of Health (2004) *The National Service Framework for Mental Health – Five years on* at **www.dh.gov.uk/en/Publicationsandstatistics**

Department of Health (2004) Core Document, National Service Framework for Children, Young People and Maternity Services at **https://www.gov.uk/government/uploads/system/uploads/attachment_data/file/199952/National_Service_Framework_for_Children_Young_People_and_Maternity_Serv.**

Department of Health (2006) White Paper – Our health, our care, our say: A new direction for community services. 30 January.

Department of Health (2006) *Mental Health Bill 2006: Regulatory Impact Assessment.* London: Department of Health.

Department of Health (2007) *Mental Health Bill: Amending the Mental Health Act 1983.* London: Department of Health.

Department of Health (2007) MHA 2007 Overview Nov 2007 at **www.dh.gov.uk/en/ policyandguidance/Heathandsocialcare topics/Mental health**

Department of Health (2007) *Mental Health Act 1983 Draft Revised Code of Practice* (2007) Para 4.4. London: DoH.

Department of Health (2008) *Refocusing the Care Programme Approach: Best practice guidance.* London: DoH.

Department of Health (2009) *Delivering Race Equality in Mental Health Care; A review by Melba Wilson, London* at **www.nmhdu.org.uk/silo/files/delivering-race-equality-in-mental-health-care-a-review.pdf**

Department of Health (2009) *Living Well With Dementia: A national dementia strategy.* London: DoH.

Department of Health (2010) *New Horizons: A shared vision for mental health.* London: DoH.

Department of Health (2011) *No Health Without Mental Health: A cross government mental health outcomes strategy for people of all ages.*

Department of Health (2011) *Me and My Schools: Findings from the national evaluation of targeted mental health in schools* at **www.gov.uk/government/uploads/system/uploads/attachment_data/ file/184060/DFE-RR177.pdf**

Department of Health (2012) *Children and Young People's Health Outcomes Strategy* at **www.gov.uk/ government/uploads/system/uploads/attachment_data/file/216853/CYP-Mental-Health.pdf**

Department of Health (2012) *No Health without Mental Health: Implementation Strategy.* London: DoH.

Department of Health (2013) *Improving Children and Young People's Health Outcomes: A system wide response.*

Department of Health, Social Services and Public Safety (2012) *Delivering the Bamford Vision: The response of Northern Ireland Executive to the Bamford review of Mental Health and Learning Disability. Action Plan 2012-2015* at **www.dhsspsni.gov.uk**

DfES (2003) *Every Child Matters: change for children* **http://webarchive.nationalarchives.gov. uk/20130401151715/https://www.education.gov.uk/publications/eOrderingDownload/ DfES10812004.pdf**

Dogra, N., Parkin, A., Gale, F. and Frake, C. (2001) *A Multidisciplinary Handbook of Child and Adolescent Mental Health for Front Line Professionals.* London: Jessica Kingsley.

Dominelli, L. (1988) *Anti–Racist Social Work. A challenge for white practitioners and educators.* Basingstoke: Macmillan.

Double, D. (2006) *Critical Psychiatry: Limits of madness.* New York. Palgrave Macmillan.

Eastman, N. (1995) Antitherapeutic community mental health law. *British Medical Journal*, 310, 1081–2.

Eldergill, A. (1997) *Mental Health Law Review Tribunals: Law and practice.* Sweet and Maxwell: London.

Epstein, S. (1983) Natural healing processes of the mind, in J. Newton (1988) *Preventing Mental Illness*, London: Routledge.

European Commission (2005) Green Paper – Improving the mental health of the population: Towards a strategy on mental health for the European Union.

Fennell, P. (2007) *Mental Health: The new law.* Bristol: Jordan Publishing.

Fernado, S. (1999) Ethnicity and mental health, in M. Ulas and A. Connor, *Mental Health and Social Work.* London: Jessica Kinglsey.

Findings (2004) *Understanding What Children Say About Living with Domestic Violence, Parental Substance Misuse or Parental Health Problems.* York: JRF.

Finzen, A. (2002) in S. Priebe and M. Slade *Evidence in Mental Health Care.* Hove: Brunner-Routledge.

Fish, J. (2012) *Social Work and Lesbian, Gay, Bisexual and Trans People: Making a difference.* Policy Press: Bristol.

Fox, C. and Hawton, K. (2004) *Deliberate Self-Harm in Adolescence.* London: Jessica Kingsley.

Fox, P., Caraher, M. and Baker, H. (2001) *Promoting Student Mental Health.* Mental Health Foundation Update 2,11.

Frangou, S. and Bryne, P. (2000) How to manage the first episode of schizophrenia. *British Medical Journal*, 321 (7260): 522.

Fulford, K.W.M. (2004a) Ten principles of values-based practice (VBP), in Radden (ed.) *Companion to the Philosophy of Psychiatry.* New York: Oxford University Press.

Fulford, K.W.M. (2004b) *Values in Mental Health Services*, in Mental Health Act Commission Tenth Biennial Report 2001–3. Norwich: Stationery Office.

Gilbert, P. (2003) *The Value of Everything: Social work and its importance in the field of mental health.* Lyme Regis: Russell House Publishing.

Glover, K. in T. Bassett and S. Cuthbert (2000) *Certificate in Community Mental Health.* Student's workbook. Southampton: Ashford Press.

Goffman, E. (1961) *Asylums.* London: Penguin.

Golightley, T.M. (1985) *If Only They Would Listen: The case for a community orientated mental health service.* Lincoln: University of Lincoln.

Gomm, R. (2004) *Social Research Methodology: Critical introduction.* Basingstoke: Palgrave Macmillan.

Gottlieb, B. (ed) (1981) *Social Networks and Social Support.* London: Sage.

Gould, M. (2008) Will community treatment orders work? *Health Service Journal* accessed 23 March 2008 from **www.hsj.co.uk/insideknowledge/2008/01/will_community_treatment_orders_ work.html**

Gregory, M.J. and Thompson, A. (2013) From here to recovery: one service user's journey through a mental health crisis: some reflections on experience, policy and practice. *Journal of Social Work Practice: Psychotherapeutic Approaches in Health, Welfare and the Community*, DOI: 10.1080/02650533.2013.802678 .

Griffiths, R. (1988) *Community Care: Agenda for action.* London: HMSO.

Hart, A., Blincow, D. and Thomas, H. (2007) *Resilient Therapy, Working with Children and Familes.* London: Routledge.

Health Advisory Service (1994) *Suicide Prevention: The challenge confronted.* London: HMSO.

Health Advisory Service (1995) *Child and Adolescent Mental Health Services – Together We Stand.* London: HMSO.

Health Advisory Service (2001) *Substance Misuse and Mental Health Comorbidity (Dual Diagnosis): Standards for Mental Health Services.* London: HAS.

HCPC (2012) *Guidence on Conduct and Ethics for Students.* Health Care Professions Council: London.

Hewitt, D. (2005) An inconvenient mirror – do we already have the next Mental Health Act. *Journal of Mental Health Law*, November, 138–49.

Hewitt, D. (2007) *The Nearest Relative Handbook.* London: Jessica Kingsley.

Hines, S. (2007) *TransForming Gender: Transgender practices of identity intimacy and care.* Bristol: Policy Press.

Horner, N. (2003) *What is Social Work? Context and perspectives.* Exeter: Learning Matters.

Hothersall, S. and Maas-Lowit, M. (eds) (2010) *Need, Risk and Protection in Social Work Practice.* Exeter: Learning Matters.

Howe, D. (1998) Relationship-based thinking and practice in social work. *Journal of Social Work Practice*, 12: 45–56.

Health & Social Care Information Centre (hscic) (Oct 2013) *Inpatients Formally Detained in Hospitals Under the Mental Health Act 1983 and Patients Subject to Supervised Community Treatment, England – 2012–2013, Annual figures* at **www.hscic.gov.uk/catalogue/PUB12503**

Huxley, P. (1985) *Social Work Practice in Mental Health.* Aldershot: Gower.

Huxley, P. (2002) Evidence in social care, in S. Priebe and M. Slade, *Evidence in Mental Health Care.* Hove: Brunner-Routledge.

James, J. (2003) *Seeing Through Walls: A report on social inclusion in practice based on the findings of the Social Inclusion Mapping Exercise.* Durham: Northern Centre for Mental Health.

John, M. and Trevithick, P. (2012) Psychodynamic thinking in social work practice, in P. Stepney and D. Ford (eds) *Social Work Models, Methods and Theories* (Second edition). Lyme Regis: Russell House.

Johns, R. (2003) *Using the Law in Social Work.* Exeter: Learning Matters.

Jones, K. (1972) *A History of the Mental Health Services.* London: Routledge and Kegan Paul.

Jones, K. (1993) *Asylums and After: A revised history of the mental health services from the early 18th century to the 1900s.* London: Athlone Press.

Jones, K. et al. (1985) *After Hospital: A study of long term psychiatric patients in York.* York: York District Health Authority.

Jones, R. (2012) *Mental Health Act Manual* (15th edition). London: Sweet and Maxwell.

Joseph Rowntree Foundation (2004) *Mental Health Service Users and their Involvement in Risk Assessment and Management.* York: JRF ref. 414.

Kalfi, Y. and Torabi, M. (1996) The Role of Parental 'Expressed Emotion' in Relapse of Schizophrenia. *Iran Journal of Medicine*: 21(1 72): 46.

Keating, F. and Robertson, D. (2002) Breaking the circles of fear: a review of mental health services to African and Caribbean communities. *Your Shout: Mental Health Promotion*, Issue 4. 18–19.

Kim, W.J. (1995) A training guideline of cultural competence for child and adolescent psychiatric residencies. *Child Psychiatry and Human Development* 26: 2, 125–36.

Kitwood, T (1997) *Dementia Reconsidered: The person comes first (Rethinking ageing).* Open University Press: Buckingham.

Kreitman, N. (1997) *Parasuicide.* Chichester: Wiley.

Laing, R.D. (1985) *Wisdom, Madness and Folly. The making of a psychiatrist.* Basingstoke: Macmillan.

Lamb, H.R. et al. (2002) *The Police and Mental Health*, Psychiatric Services 2002; doi: 10.1176/appi. ps.53.10.1266 available at **http://journals.psychiatryonline.org/article.aspx?Volume=53&page=1 266&journalID=18**

Langan, J. and Lindow, V. (2004) *Living with Risk: Mental health service user involvement in risk assessment and management.* Bristol: Policy Press.

Leader, D. (2012) *What is Madness?* Penguin Books: St. Ives.

Leff, J., Kuipers, K. and Lam, D. (2002) *Family Work for Schizophrenia* (2nd edition). London: Royal College of Psychiatrists.

Lloyd, E. (1999) *What Works in Parenting Education.* Barnardos. Summary available at **www.barnardos.org.uk/what_works_in_parenting_education__1999_-_summary.pdf**

Low, J. (2004) *Lay acquiescence to medical dominance in assessing the efficacy of alternative and complementary therapies: reflections on the active citizenship thesis.* Paper presented to the European Sociological Association Symposium on Professions, Social Inclusion and Citizenship. Lincoln: University of Lincoln.

Lyall, J. (2006) The Struggle for Cultural Competence. The *Guardian*, Wednesday, 12 April 2006.

MacLean, M. (2004) *Together and Apart: Children and parents experiencing divorce.* York: JRF (Foundations series).

Mckeown, M. and Mercer, D. (1998) Language, race and forensic psychiatry, in T. Mason and C. Mercer, (eds) *Critical Perspectives in Forensic Care.* Basingstoke: Macmillan.

Meehan, J. et al. (2006) Suicide in mental health in-patients and within 3 months of discharge. National clinical survey. *British Journal of Psychiatry,* Feb, 188: 129–34.

Menninger, K. (1963) *The Vital Balance: The life process in mental health and illness.* London: Viking Press.

Mental Capacity Act Code of Practice (2007) London: The Stationery Office.

Mental Health Alliance (3 July 2007) *Mental Health Bill remains a missed opportunity for humane and progressive legislation,* Press Release.

Mental Health Act Commission (MHAC) (1998) Written submission to House of Lords. In Shaw, I., Middleton, H. and Cohen, J. (2007) *Understanding Treatment without Consent.* Aldershot: Ashgate.

Mental Health Act Commission (1999–2001) *Ninth Biennial Report.* London: Stationery Office.

Mental Health Foundation (1999) *The Big Picture: Promoting children and young people's mental health.* London: Mental Health Foundation.

Mental Health Law online (2013) *Judgment in Ian Brady Tribunal* at **www.mentalhealthlaw.co.uk/ Re_Ian_Brady_%282013%29_MHLO_89_%28FTT%29**

Mischon, J. (2000) Report of the independent inquiry team into the care and treatment of Daniel Joseph. Sutton and Wandsworth Health Authority and Lambeth, Southwark and Lewisham Health Authority.

Modestein and Schwarzenbach (1992) Effect of psycho–pharmacotherapy on suicide risk in discharged psychiatric patients, Acta Psychiatrica Scandinavia in C. Pritchard (1995) *Suicide – The Ultimate Rejection.* Buckingham: Open University Press.

Moore, M. et al. (2009) Explaining the rise in antidepressant prescribing: a descriptive study using the general practice research database. *British Medical Journal,* 2009; 339: b3999.

Moss, S et al. (2000) Psychiatric symptoms in adults with learning disability and challenging behaviour. *British Journal of Pyschiatry,* November 2000 177: 452–56; doi:10.1192/bjp.177.5.452.

Nathan, J. and Webber, M. (2010) Mental health social work and the bureau-medicalisation of mental health care: Identity in a changing world. *Journal of Social Work Practice,* Vol. 24 , issue 1 , 2010, Taylor and Francis.

National Collaborating Centre for Mental Health (2013) *Psychosis and Schizophrenia in Children and Young: Recognition and management.* National Clinical Guideline Number 155, National Institute for Health and Care Excellence.

Nazroo, J. (1999) *Ethnicity and Mental Health.* London: Policy Studies Institute.

Neustatter, A. (2003) Changing shapes, in *Young Minds Magazine,* No 68.

Newman, T. and Blackburn, S. (2002) *Transitions in the Lives of Children and Young People: Resilience factors.* Barnardo's Policy, Research and Influencing Unit: Scottish Executive Education Department.

Newton, J. (1988) *Preventing Mental Illness.* London: Routledge.

NIMHE (2003) Inside outside: improving mental health services for black and minority ethnic communities in England at **www.devon.gov.uk/inside_outside.pdf** (accessed 25 May 2011).

NIMHE (2006) National Suicide Prevention Strategy for England: Annual Report on Progress 2005. Care Service Improvement Partnership: Leeds.

Office of the Public Guardian (2007) *Mental Capacity Act Code of Practice* at **www.justice.gov.uk/ protecting-the-vulnerable/mental-capacity-act**

Office for National Statistics (1999) *Social Trends no 31* at **www.ons.gov.uk/ons/rel/social-trends-rd/social-trends/index.html**

O'Hagan, K. (ed) (1996) *Competence in Social Work Practice.* London: Jessica Kingsley.

O'Hagan, K. (2001) *Cultural Competence in the Caring Professions*. London: Jessica Kingsley.

O'Sullivan, T. (1999) *Decision Making in Social Work*. Basingstoke: Macmillan.

Obafunwa, J.O. and Busuttil, A. (1994) Clinical contact preceding suicide, in C. Pritchard (1995) *Suicide – The Ultimate Rejection*. Buckingham: Open University Press.

Oliver, M. (1996) *Understanding Disability: from theory to practice*. Basingstoke: Macmillan.

Onyett, S. (1992) *Case Management in Mental Health*. Cheltenham: Stanley Thornes.

Orbach, S. (1986) *Hunger Strike*. London: Penguin.

Our Health, Our Care, Our Say: A new direction for community services. White Paper accessible at **www.dh.gov.uk/ourhealthourcareoursay** (accessed 25 May 2011)

Parker, J. and Bradley, G. (2003) *Social Work Practice: Assessment, planning, intervention and review*. Exeter: Learning Matters.

Patel, K. et al. (2003) *Engaging and Changing: Developing effective policy for the care and treatment of black and minority ethnic detained patients*. London: DoH.

Pearce, J. (1999) Collaboration between the NHS and Social Services in the provision of child and adolescent mental health services: a personal view. *Child Psychology and Psychiatry Review*, 4: 4, 150–3.

Pharoah, F.M., Mari, J.J. and Steiner, D. (2000) *American Journal of Psychiatry*, 153, 607–17 in the Cochrane Library issue 3, 2002, Oxford update software.

Pilgrim, D. and Rogers, A. (1999) *A Sociology of Mental Health and Illness* (2nd edition). Buckingham: Open University Press.

Pollack, W. (1999) *Real Boys*. New York: Henry Holt.

Poole, D.L. (1998) Politically correct or culturally competent. *Health and Social Work*, 23 (3) 163–6.

Practice Direction First-tier Tribunal. Health, Education and Social Care Chamber. Mental Health Cases, 2013 available at: **www.judiciary.gov.uk/Resources/JCO/Documents/Practice%20Directions/ Tribunals/statements-in-mental-health-cases-hesc-28102013.pdf**

Priebe, S. and Slade, M. (2002) *Evidence in Mental Health Care*. Hove: Brunner-Routledge.

Prins, H. (1999) *Will They Do It Again?: Risk assessment and management in criminal justice and psychiatry*. London: Routledge.

Pritchard, C. (1995) *Suicide – The Ultimate Rejection*. Buckingham: Open University Press.

Ramon, S. (2001) Opinions and dilemmas facing British mental health social work, in J. Tew, Going social: championing a holistic model of mental distress within professional education, *Social Work Education*, Vol 21, No 2, 2002.

Ray, M., Pugh, R. with Roberts, D. and Beech, B. (2008) *Social Care Institute for Excellence research briefing 26: mental health and social work* at **www.scie.org.uk/publications/briefings/briefing26/ index.asp** (accessed 25 May 2011)

Red Manual Code of Practice (2004) *Section D:10 working with parents with mental health problems*. Lincoln: Lincolnshire County Council.

Rethink Sane and Zito Trust (2003) Behind Closed Doors: The current state and future of acute mental health care in the UK. London: *Rethink* at **www.mentalhealthshop.org/promotional_items** (accessed 25 May 2011)

Ridgeway, S.M. (1997) Deaf people and psychological health – some preliminary findings. *Deaf Worlds*, Issue 1, Vol 13, 9–17.

Rikken, M. (1995) A preventive mental health programme for children of parents with mental disorders, in D. Trent and A. Reed (1995) *Promotion of Mental Health*. Aldershot: Ashgate.

Ritchie, J.H., Dick D. and Lingham, R. (1994) *The Report of the Inquiry into the Care and Treatment of Christopher Clunis*. London: HMSO.